Healing the Planet

ONE PATIENT AT A TIME

A Primer in Environmental Medicine

Jozef J. Krop,
MD, FAAEM

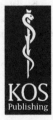

KOS
Publishing

Healing the Planet One Patient at a Time:
A Primer in Environmental Medicine

National Library of Canada Cataloguing in Publication

Krop, Jozef J., 1944–
  Healing the planet: one patient at a time : a primer in environmental medicine / Jozef J. Krop.

Includes bibliographical references and index.
ISBN-10: 0-9731945-0-2   ISBN-13: 978-0-9731945-0-0

  1. Environmental toxicology. 2. Environmental health. 3. Environmentally induced diseases. I. Title.

RA565.K76 2002   615.9'02   C2002-905674-8

Sixth printing, 2013

Cover and text design/layout, print production: WeMakeBooks.ca

Photo credit: Arne Jacenty, AJ Photographic

Printed and bound in Canada.

Text pages printed on recycled paper

Published and distributed by KOS Publishing Inc.
1997 Beechgrove Road,
Alton, ON Canada L0N 1A0
Tel/Fax (519) 927-1049
Quantity discounts available

Table of Contents

Publisher's Preface to the Second Printing

The first printing of this book, November 2002, was quickly sold out, making a second printing necessary eight months later. It is a matter of special satisfaction to me personally, that while sold in major bookstores everywhere, most were sold in doctors' offices. This means that this book is primarily in the hands of patients whose doctors work *with* them.

For more than two decades, Dr. Krop's name has been associated in North America with the politics of medicine. He is best known for his role in helping to launch the popularly known "Kwinter Bill" (after Ontario's Liberal MPP Monte Kwinter), which enshrined patient's freedom of choice in the Medicine Act of Ontario in 2000 (see Ontario Hansard of August 28, 1991). Dr. Krop also contributed, in the early 1980s to the World Commission on the Environment (the *Brundtland Report*), and his practice was used by the Ontario government to begin the process of establishing guidelines for dealing with environmental causes of illness (the 1985 *Thomson Report*). He also participated in various university and federal government-sponsored efforts to raise awareness of the environment's impact on population health. In the 1980s he was a co-founder, and for many years served as the secretary of the Canadian Society for Environmental Medicine.

As is the fate of many pioneers, he spent more than a decade defending environmental medicine in a disciplinary trial initiated against him by the Ontario medical licensing authority, the *College of Physicians and Surgeons of Ontario*. The CPSO based their prosecution not on patient complaints (there were none), adverse treatment outcome (they admitted all files studied showed the patients had improved), but alleged that practicing environmental medicine "lacked acceptable scientific evidence"[1]. The CPSO then ensured that such scientific evidence appeared indeed to be missing by totally ignoring its existence when handing down their final 1999 Decision. Many of those hundreds of scientific articles, all from the mainstream medical journals, provided by the defense lawyers during the trial, are now part of the reference section in this book. Of course, this throwback to medieval doctrinal wars and its legal instrument, the Inquisition, begins to make some sense when one realizes that the majority of CPSO council members are either directly or indirectly connected to the pharmaceutical and pesticide industry.

Dr. Krop's trial is legally, politically, and medically one of the great scandals in medical history. His patients and supporters fortunately believed in this cause and footed most of the defense bill which, over that long decade of the trial, reached almost Can. $2 million. However, due this immense effort and the involvement of so many first class lawyers, the legal profession became sensitized to the abuse of process and law the CPSO and other regulatory bodies committed without ever being checked. Today there are many lawyers working for many more innovative doctors and defending medicine properly. Before the Krop case few lawyers and judges knew just how deep the rot ran. Those who want to know more about this story and the world-wide battle for Environmental Medicine, may want to read **Malice in Medicine—***The 14-Year Trial of Environmental Medicine Physician* **Dr. Jozef Krop** written by me and due to be published in 2004.

This book is a primer preface in environmental medicine. It is unique among the many excellent books currently available on many aspects of health and environment because this one is meant for *both* patients and doctors. Knowing that patients are intelligent people who can understand anything in medicine if the courtesy of full explanation is offered, Dr. Krop includes in this book the complete treatment protocols which the reader can take to his or her doctor to study. These protocols are supported by an exhaustive medical bibliography intended especially for those Doubting Thomases who are willing to examine widely-held prejudices against environmental medicine and are willing to consider seriously its claim to be able to help those many illnesses standard medicine calls idiopathic, i.e. cause unknown. Every year more and more research is published showing;

that what was once considered an idiopathic illness is now well understood as environmentally and nutritionally mediated. Water, air and soil polluted with neuro-toxins and carcinogens, and nutrient-deficient processed food laced with endocrine disrupters and pesticides cause or trigger virtually all modern epidemics, such as asthma, chronic fatigue, most neurological diseases, Parkinson's, Alzheimer's, allergies, osteoporosis, attention deficit disorder and many psychiatric conditions, cardiovascular disease, depression, and the greatest scourge of our time—cancer.[2]

Since *Healing The Planet Once Patient At A Time* appeared last year, Dr. Krop was reprimanded in September 2003 for practicing medicine lacking scientific proof—as interpreted by Ontario's medical licensing authorities. Dr. Krop is free to practice; the CPSO's "victory" is more of an embarrassment than a triumph and will serve to help spread the word about environmental medicine rather than deter its practice. For purposes of comparison, the reader may be interested in how the CPSO's monumental ignorance and arrogance measure up to current developments in environmental and nutritional medicine. This is merely a sample—a complete list is beyond the scope of this preface. Indeed, a great shift in understanding is taking place in medicine, which will, no doubt, eventually leave the corporately contaminated regulatory authorities and medical practitioners in the dust.

- The December 2000 health-freedom amendment to the Ontario Medicine Act sponsored by Liberal MPP Monte Kwinter and whose wording he took from the 1988 international Helsinki Accord on Human Rights, has taken on a lifer of its own. Similar bills are now being sponsored by provincial legislators in Saskatchewan, Manitoba, and Quebec. It already exists in British Columbia; Alberta was the first to make it law.

- Following the Canadian Supreme Court's Hudson Decision of 2002 on the right to pass local by-laws against pesticide use, an immense public campaign brought about in March this year the passage of an anti-pesticide law for the whole Province of Quebec where its cosmetic use will be phased out completely. Within a decade we may have epidemiological evidence that in Quebec population health has markedly improved, compared to the rest of Canada.

- The World Health Organization recently published a consensus report on the need to reduce drastically the use of refined sugar, remove vending pop machines from school cafeterias, and reduce the amount of sugar in processed foods. The sugar industry was infuriated and demanded from the WHO's Director General, Gro Brundtland, that this report be withdrawn, threatening that otherwise the industry would see to it that the WHO's annual financial contribution from the United States government would be withheld. Dr. Brundtland responded by publishing both the report and the threats.[3] Incidentally, in 1993 the CPSO reprimanded Toronto's Dr. Carolyn Dean for warning against the intake of too much sugar while being interviewed on the Dini Petti television show—the warning was specific to diabetic patients and warned also against high sugar intake as causing diabetes. A complaint by Canada's Sugar Institute had initiated this disciplinary investigation on the grounds that there was "no scientific basis" for such a claim against refined sugar. This casts an interesting light on where the CPSO gets its scientific advice.[4]

- Commencing in April of 2002, the Canadian Medical Association's official journal, the CMAJ, published a six-part series on environment and health covering the proper way to take an exposure history (April 16), the effects of outdoor pollution (April 30), recognizing and treating lead exposure (May 14), management and prevention regarding pesticides (May 28), the health effects of persistent organic pollutants (June 11), and understanding carbon monoxide poisoning (June 25). The authors are leading experts in those areas and teach at Canada's medical school. Most noteworthy is the fact that the references and research sources provided in those articles were almost all also those Dr. Krop's defense lawyers had given to the CPSO during his trial.[5]

- In October 2003 the Ontario College of Family Physicians hosted its first medical conference on Environmental Medicine and participating physicians received full continuing study credits from the Ontario Medical Association.

- At the beginning of this year, Canada's Ministry of Human Resources responded to requests for help from advocacy groups working with victims of Multiple Chemical Sensitivity (MCS). RAINET (Research, Advocacy.) approached the Minister, the Hon. Jane Stewart and provided case histories of individuals who were totally disabled by exposure to certain toxic chemicals, but were denied CPP and other applicable benefits solely on the basis of an MCS diagnosis. A review was initiated and MCS is now in the process of being included for CPP benefits. The core problem in the case of Dr. Krop before the CPSO was the diagnosis of MCS which was rejected as being "scientifically invalid" the same month, June 1999, when the international consensus statement on MCS as a valid diagnosis was published by the National Institutes of Health in the USA.[6]

- One of the treatments for which the CPSO condemned Dr. Krop is a desensitization procedure for environmental and food allergies through the use of sub-lingual drops. (See footnote no. 1 for Internet access to the CPSO decision). In April 2002, 4 months after the CPSO verdict, the World Health Organization published a report, based on the review by 34 internationally recruited allergists, stating that this treatment should be considered the treatment of choice.[7]

- The Ontario Human Rights Commission wrote in April of this year to Ontario's Minister of Health, the Hon. Tony Clement, instructing him that in the event of spraying for West Nile Virus being considered, the Minister has the obligation to protect people with chemical sensitivities and to ensure they receive medical care if affected by the spraying. The federal government made a similar statement.[8]

- A few years ago, the American Preventive Medical Association (APMA) sued the United Stated Food and Drug Administration (FDA) because of that agency's persecution of anybody making any health claims for vitamins and other neutraceuticals. The case was decided in favor of the APMA, but in clear defiance of the court order, the FDA continued to harass doctors and neutraceutical companies. This year in May, another court case was decided once again in favor of the APMA, and now the FDA obeyed the court. Health claims for all antioxidants (such as Vitamins C and E), Folic Acid, various fiber supplements and Saw Palmetto are now appearing on supplement bottles.

- In an abrupt turn-around only comparable to a conversion experience, one of the world's leading experts in nutrition and health, Bruce Ames of the University of California at Berkeley published a comprehensive review article in April 2002 in which he asserts that Linus Pauling was right all along. Coming from Bruce Ames, that's a bit like the leader of the Alliance Party joining the NDP. Shortly thereafter, the Journal of the American Medical Association published in June 2002 two articles, which conclude that everybody needs to take vitamin and mineral supplements to prevent chronic disease, and that no diet provides enough of the nutrients needed for basic good health and to prevent chronic illness later in life.[9]

- One of the sections in Dr. Krop's book deals with autism, its causes and treatment for which he provides the appropriate protocols. Due to the efforts of Congressman Dan Burton in the USA, whose grandson became autistic after being vaccinated for Mumps Measles and Rubella, the vaccine industry has been forced this spring to remove the offending mercury used as a preservative in vaccines.[10]

All these developments in such a short period of time led Dr. Krop to observe jokingly, "If we wait long enough, they'll make intravenous vitamin C the standard of treatment for SARS."

While all these shifts in understanding are very encouraging indeed, this is not the time for complacency. Nutritional and environmental medicine is still under attack because its claims, research and success are a fundamental threat to the pharmaceutical and pesticide industry. As Cornell University's ecologist and cancer expert Sandra Steingraber has pointed out, the world's economy is "chemically addicted",[11] and that the health of the world is endangered by nothing as much as by that "toxic trespass"[12] committed without our knowledge, and often against our will, by a chemical industry in conscious disregard of the biological requirements and biochemical integrity of humanity. Similarly, the drug industry's products are now, due to their serious adverse "side"-effects, considered to be the second most frequent cause of death[13]. Clearly, we have a long way to go before doctors and patients become free from quick-fix delusions and understand that health is a matter of prevention, proper nutrition, and therapies that work *with* nature.

The fact that a book such as this one sells well and that all of the above (and much more) is published by the mainstream medical journals, and supported by standard national and international medical organizations, indicates that a big change is happening. People are taking charge and thinking critically. Fortunately, the Internet ensures that information cannot be buried as it used to be and high-speed communication has created something of a level playing field for health activists.

Yet, there are many actions still ongoing which are of grave importance and require our determined support. For example, the international battle being waged against CODEX, the international regulatory body controlled by the pharmaceutical companies; it seeks to make all neutraceuticals available by prescription only. Another important and parallel cause is that championed by Canadian federal MPP Dr. J. Lunney's and his courageous and timely effort (Bill C 420) which seeks to prevent Health Canada from gaining control over food supplements; in view of Health Canada's track record with regard to drug approval and its efforts to prevent information on food safety from becoming publicly known, they certainly don't need to control neutraceuticals as well.[14]

In antiquity it was believed that the source of medical knowledge was divine and that the ability to practice medicine was a gift granted by the god of medicine himself, Asklepios. By definition gods are immortal and divine truth cannot be destroyed and, therefore, will once again make us free.

Helke Ferrie, Publisher
Kos Publishing Inc. • *Books on Medicine that Works!*
Alton, Ontario, Canada   August 2003

ENDNOTES

1 CPSO Decision on Dr. Krop, December 23, 1998, available on their website: **www.cpso.on.ca**

2 One of the best sources for information on the environmental component or cause of any disease is found in *Environmental Health Perspectives*, a medical journal published monthly by the National Institutes of Health and Harvard University's School of Public Health; available on-line.

3 *The Medical Post*, May 13, 2003.

4 The College of Physicians and Surgeons of Ontario reprimanded Dr. Carolyn Dean on April 29, 1993, based on a complaint filed by Sandra Marsden of the Sugar Institute of Canada; the complaint was filed, as stated in the admonishment document, because Dr. Dean had spoken about the *dangers of refined sugar intake by diabetics on a television show aired on December 11, 1990. The reprimand states: "The respondent made inaccurate and misleading statements addressing health issues related to sugar and sugar substitutes ... which tended to potentially arouse concern in the viewing public . The Committee believes the respondent expressed opinions which appeared to be exaggerated with respect to the relationship between sugar and diabetes, infection, osteoporosis, hyperactivity and addiction."* This amazing nonsense, unsupported by any published medical evidence, was signed by Dr. D.M.C. Walker, then the CPSO president and now the Dean of medicine at Queen's University in Kingston, Ontario. In her defence, prior to this admonishment, Dr. Dean had submitted more than 200 citations from the then current, standard, peer-reviewed medical literature on sugar and sugar substitutes upon which her remark on television had been based. This material is not even mentioned in the admonishment.

5 CMAJ, Vol. 166, April 16 through June 25, 2002

6 *Archives of Environmental Health*, vol. 54, No. 3, pp. 147–149, June 1999

7 See summary in *Scientific American*, April 2002, p. 26, "Drink Your Shots" by B. Goodman

8 Letter from the Ontario Human Rights Commission, dated April 16, 2003, signed by Chief Commissioner Keith C. Norton, addressed to the Hon. Tony Clement, Ontario's Minister of Health; the legal basis cited is the *Ontario Human Rights Code*, Section 29 and the Policy *and Guidelines on Disability and the Duty to Accommodate*

9 The *American Journal of Clinical Nutrition*, April 2002 and *Journal of the American Medical Association*, June 19, 2002

10 For a copy of my article on autism contact Vitality magazine at 416-964-0528; it provides the historical, legal and treatment information. See also Autism Canada Foundation, P.O. Box 366, Bothwell, ON, N0P 1C0, Telephone: (519) 695-5858, Fax: (519) 695-5757, visit **www.autismcanada.org**. Dr. J. Bradstreet's institute can be reached via **www.icdrc.org** and **www.autismresearchinstitute.com**

11 S. Steingraber, Living *Downstream*: An Ecologist Looks at Cancer, 2nd ed. 1999

12 S. Steingraber in the upcoming documentary, *If You Love Our Children*, sponsored by The National Film Board of Canada.

13 J.S. Cohen, *Overdose: The Case Against the Drug Companies*, Tarcher-Putnam, 2001. J. Robinson, *Prescription Games*, McLelland & Stewart, Toronto, 2001. T.J. Moore, *Prescription for Disaster*, Simon & Schuster, 1998. J. Glenmullen, *Prozac Backlash*, Touchstone Books, 2000. Canadian Assoctaion of University teachers, *The Olivieri Report*, Lorimer, 20021.

14 To help stop the international efforts under the United nations' CODEX ALIMENTARIUS to restrict the availability of vitamins and supplements, contact the worldwide effort being coordinated by Dr. Matthias Rath in Germany at **ttp://www4.dr-rath-foundation.org/ features/codex_wto.html**. In Canada, Dr. James Lunney introduced Bill C 420 for the same purpose, to maintain freedom of choice for Canadians. The bill is available on **www.parl.gc.ca/37/2parlbus/chambus/house/bills/private/C-420I/C-420cover-E.html** and you can contact your own MP and express your support for this bill.

Preface

Dr. Jozef Krop is a citizen of Canada. I am a citizen of the United States. Although we may reside in different countries, when it comes to health and medicine, our problems are the same. Both countries suffer from the same pollution, and from a similar Medical-Pharmaceutical monopoly in the treatment of disease.

Several years ago, I spent the night at the home of a friend. That same night, Edgar Mitchell a former astronaut, also stayed at my friend's house. The next morning they were making a film in the front yard of my friend's home.

Ed Mitchell sat beside a large globe of the world. He said, "As we were traveling towards the moon, our crew of three realized that we had to work together with our limited space, our limited resources and our limited waste disposal system in that spaceship if the flight was to be successful and we were to survive."

He said, "I looked out that little window and saw that beautiful blue and white ball we call Earth. Then a strange thing happened. All of a sudden I realized that that blue and white ball we call Earth was a spaceship just as surely as was the one in which we were traveling. And it had limited space, limited resources and a limited waste disposal system just as surely as did ours.

But whereas the three of us were working together to try to bring the flight through successfully, the crew on spaceship Earth was not doing the same."

How right he was, as we pollute our planet with insecticides, pesticides and manufactured chemicals of all types.

We not only pollute our planet, we also pollute our bodies with cigarette smoke in our lungs; chemicals in our clothing, furniture and carpets; mercury in our teeth; and chemicals and pollutants in the air we breathe, the water we drink and the food we eat.

When George Washington became ill, he was treated with bloodletting and mercury, one of the most poisonous materials known. He died.

Now we no longer treat people with mercury. We simply put it in people's teeth, so that they can absorb this powerful poison day and night, whether they are sick or well.

We no longer bleed cancer patients. We simply inject into their blood a poison so strong that patients' hair falls off, and those administering it dare not get any of it on their skin.

Conventional medicine may not have changed that much, but people have started to change since the time of George Washington. People are also starting to rebel. Many of them are no longer willing to submit to the poisonous treatments advocated by many conventional doctors. More and more people are buying organic produce, and more of them are buying bottled water to avoid the chlorine and poisonous fluoride added to the water by many water treatment plants.

All through history, science has ridiculed and persecuted those who have challenged the prevailing beliefs and systems. We can thank God for the Galileos and the Darwins. And yes, we can thank God for Jozef Krop and other courageous individuals who are willing to challenge the system.

Today the practice of toxic medicine is even more entrenched than at the time of George Washington. Billions and billions of dollars of profits are at stake. It is already obvious that this powerful monopoly will do whatever it has to do to protect its turf and profits.

But all through history, in the final analysis, the people have prevailed. And now a revolution has begun. People are starting to take command of their health with decisions on the food, water and air they consume. More and more are refusing the toxic treatments frequently prescribed by conventional doctors. And more and more they want to learn for themselves how to keep healthy and avoid toxicity, whether it comes from the environment or is administered by a doctor.

That is why this book and the life and work of Joe Krop are so important. Although attacked and scorned by the medical-pharmaceutical monopoly with their toxic treatments, Joe Krop has refused to buckle.

This book is a step into the present for those who think their health is more important than the income and profits of a medical-pharmaceutical monopoly.

I am thankful to God for people like Joe Krop and for books such as this. I urge those who wish to remain healthy or recover if they become ill to read and study this book and to become part of this revolutionary movement that is finally starting to take place. It has been over two hundred years since the death of George Washington. It is about time that we recognize that the consumption of chemicals, toxins and poisons is not the way to stay healthy or become healthy.

Berkley Bedell
Former US Congressman
Founder, National Foundation for Alternative Medicine.

This book is dedicated to my children,
Joanna, Jessica, Adam and Andrew,
as well as to all the children of the world,
born and yet to be born—
to protect them from the insidious pollutants of this world.

"Above all, do no harm."

"Medicine is not a science but an art."

"Every disease has its own nature and arises
from an external cause."

"Let food be your medicine."
—Hippocrates (c 460–c 377 B.C.)

"To understand the man we have to understand his world,
the environment he lives in."
—Aristotle (c 384–c 322 B.C.)

"The doctor of the future will give no medicine
but will interest his patients in the care of
the human frame, in diet and in the cause
and prevention of disease."
—Thomas A. Edison (1847-1931)

"Search for the cure within the cause;
the body itself is the best healer."
—Plato (c 429–c 347 B.C.)

Foreword

It is a great honour for me to prepare a foreword for this groundbreaking book by Dr. Krop. I first became acutely aware of the catastrophic effect of the environment on community health when the tragedy of the Love Canal began to unfold at Niagara Falls, New York. This toxic waste dump was officially recognized as America's first "disaster area" for pollution. Simultaneously, we saw the severe congenital deformities and diseases in babies born to former University of Buffalo students, who had been enticed to take short-term jobs at the West Valley Nuclear Reprocessing facility south of Buffalo, NY, exposing them to high doses of nuclear radiation. Although the health problem generated by West Valley were never officially admitted, the site became the first demonstration site in the United States for nuclear cleanup and radioactive waste stabilization.

We, at Roswell Park Memorial Institute, in Buffalo, New York, were called upon to help these two communities in trauma. Both community groups, with environmentally caused health problems, had self-identified their plight and the likely cause. Dr. Beverly Paigen, a toxicologist, and myself, an epidemiologist, tried to help the communities officially document the truths which they knew through their own observations. We had no idea how controversial such health assessment and professional assistance would be!

The spectre of lawsuits against the polluters rose up at every turn, and no health assessment or sensible epidemiological survey at either place was ever permitted. The barriers to understanding these phenomena varied from cutting out any interviewing or clinical components of retrospective studies, demanding data to be based on publically collected (inadequate) vital statistics to actually closing the Environmental Health Division of the Erie County Health Department, which was preparing a detailed epidemiological survey.

While I spent nine years studying the impact of ordinary diagnostic X-ray exposure on the health of a very large population followed over three years (The Tri-State Leukemia Survey), I had discovered that the whole question of exposure of the public to ionizing radiation had been relegated to the expertise of the physicists of the Manhattan project (which built the first nuclear bombs), and that it was these military participants who gave nuclear industries radiation standards which allow for routine radio nuclide emissions to the environment, and set worker standards quite high relative to observed medical problems. Then I found that physicians accepted the standards set by the military during atmospheric weapon testing as the appropriate standards for the hospital and radiology laboratories. In fact, many radiologists opposed releasing information on the harm of diagnostic X-rays because they were afraid that the public would refuse needed X-rays, making their work more difficult. Eventually I found that many other hazards to the public had the same military origin and were protected with the similar fears and secrecy.

Currently there is much concern about pesticides and organic compounds which mimic the effects of hormones. These derive historically from the large-scale separation of chlorine gas for military use in World War I, and the subsequent military production of chlorinated compounds, both organic and inorganic, culminating in the Agent Orange widely dispersed in Viet Nam. One of these chlorine compounds was chloroform, which found an early medical use as an anaesthetic, but was soon abandoned when it was found to cause liver damage. Carbon tetrachloride is another artifi-

cial chemical introduced, which we now trying to rid ourselves of by promoting "green dry cleaning" establishments. The organic chlorides, including many pesticides, are now ubiquitous around the world, and many disrupt
normal hormonal functions.

It is not surprising that thoughtful and intelligent physicians, especially
pediatricians, would see the results of these and so many other reckless
additions of hazardous substances to the biosphere. Dr. Krop is to be com-
plimented on being open to learning new ways of dealing with patients presenting with damage from these exposures. All university training claims to
promote a goal of lifetime learning, but few graduates excel in pioneering
new fields of research. Dr. Krop is also to be commended for standing up for
the truth he has found, in spite of the many serious attacks on his professional conduct from those who are not open to what is happening around
them and the new challenges to the traditional art and science of medicine.

We can expect many more challenging situations for human and community health to result from global warming, changes in land use, population growth, migration, modern forms of war, drug use, international trade
and commerce, technological changes, new ways to process food, livestock
handling, organ transplants, microbial changes, and breakdown in sanita-
tion, vaccination and insect control. Extreme weather events, such as
drought followed by torrential rain, can be expected to change survival patterns of both mosquitos and birds, and affect the life cycle of many
pathogens. Social and human activities bring us into more contact with
fragments of forest, and increase the incidence of Lyme disease and perhaps
other pathogens which we do not now expect. The climate warming trend
can mean survival of many pathogens which were previously killed off
during the winter. Who then, except the Environmental Physicians, will be
on the alert for new manifestations of illnesses with unfamiliar symptoms?

Environmental Health is not just a branch of occupational health. There
are no children in the workplace. Chronic low-dose 24-hour exposures of
children or the elderly are biologically and biochemically different from
adult male higher occupational exposures for eight hours a day, followed by

a 16-hour respite. And then we have a toxic "soup" not seen in the limited environment of the workplace, where hazards can be counted and monitored. Production agents in the workplace cost money, and so tend to be conserved. Any delving into the irresponsible abandonment of multiple forms of hazardous pollution in the living space will lead the prudent government regulators to welcome and facilitate the work of Environmental Physicians.

The road ahead will not be easy. In the struggle 150 years ago to understand germs, no one was standing there saying: "It is not MY germs causing the trouble." There were no lawsuits around the corner of every finding. Hazardous chemical materials in the environment are just as invisible as germs, and research into their action in the body no more complex than was the sorting out of pathogens which caused identifiable diseases. However, this research must be seriously undertaken!

The struggle against harmful environmental hazards and pathogens has just begun. The work of Dr. Krop is welcomed by all of us who have opened our eyes to the current suffering and the future potential of all of the changes and human interventions in our living space with its vital air, water and food.

Rosalie Bertell, PhD
International Institute of Concern for Public Health
Toronto, Canada

Acknowledgements

This book began as a practical "Ecology Guide," a handbook, a simple educational tool for my patients, soon after I started to practice environmental medicine. A great deal of thanks must go to past and current members of my staff, who put enormous effort into helping educate patients in their struggle to improve health, gathered information and helped arrange ever richer versions into a reader-friendly format. These include Wanda Wilson, Darlene Koski, Dawn Betts, Virginia Anderson, and Maureen Bot. I also wish to thank one of my many "angels," Andrew Pompa, who first suggested that the guide should be published as a book for wider distribution. Helke Ferrie, another "angel," was able to realize that idea, as well as make invaluable suggestions, reviewing, editing, recommending references and encouraging me tirelessly in all things. Thanks to everyone at Heidy Lawrance Associates, as well as to Simone Gabbay, for helping to produce this book in short order.

I am indebted to Rosalie Bertell, whom I have known for many years, and with whom I worked together on two projects associated with the International Institute of Concern for Public Health, for her input and review of the piece on nuclear radiation, an area about which most of us are woefully ignorant. Thank you to former Congressman Berkley Bedell, whose efforts, with Senator Tom Harkin, led to the creation of the Office of Alternative Medicine at the US National Institutes of Health.

A very special expression of gratitude to the many wonderful colleagues I have met over the years at the American Academy of Environmental Medicine, in particular physician mentors and now friends, Drs. John Maclennan and John Gerrard of Canada, as well as Drs. Frank Waickman, Bill Rea, John Boyles, Charlie Hinshaw, Denis Remington, Doris Rapp of the US, and especially the late Drs. Theron Randolph and Larry Dickie, true pioneers in the field. Prof. Lynn Trainor, physicist and dear friend, has been a pillar of support offering insight from the beginning, as have Drs. Lynn Marshall, William LaValley, Gerry Ross, and Roy Fox.

For their unflagging support over the past decade, I am grateful to: Helma Trass, Pat and Bruce Houghton, Diana Tuszynski, Audrey Sillick and Rena Singer-Gordon of the Environmental Health Group; Eleanor Johnston, Bruce Lofquist and Don McNicol of Citizens for Choice in Health Care; Judy Spence of EISC; Harold Dickert, Bob Ferrie, Maria French, Robert McMaster, Alex and Leslie Trass, Siegfried Gursche and Rhody Lake of *Alive Magazine;* Julia Woodford of *Vitality Magazine;* Libby Gardon of *Consumer Health Organization of Canada.* There are many others whose names may not be mentioned here, but for whose support I am nevertheless most grateful.

Thank you to my parents, simple and humble farmers, from whom I learned hard work, perseverance, and to appreciate the bounty of this good earth. Finally, thank you to my wife and closest friend of thirty years, Elizabeth, for standing beside, behind and sometimes in front of me in all my struggles, and for correcting everything I ever wrote in English.

Introduction

WHY THIS MEDICINE IS IMPORTANT

"In the middle of the twentieth century, we saw our planet from space for the first time. Historians may eventually find that this vision had a greater impact on thought than did the Copernican revolution of the sixteenth century, which upset the human self-image by revealing that the earth is not the center of the universe. From space, we see a small and fragile ball dominated not by human activity and edifice, but by patterns of clouds, oceans, greenery, and soils. Humanity's inability to fit its doings into that pattern is changing planetary systems fundamentally. Many such changes are accompanied by life-threatening hazards. This new reality, from which there is no escape, must be recognized—and managed."[1]

This is the opening statement from the Brundtland Commission's report, *Our Common Future*, the world commission report on environment and development published in 1987. All the nations of the world presented their concerns to this commission. I was among those who spoke as one representative from Canada on behalf of medicine. I spoke before the commission in 1985 about my fears as a doctor, namely that "we discuss forests, agricultural land, plant and animal life, but virtually ignore the real threat to the very existence of the human species."[2]

In 1985, those were strong words; today, neither scientists nor politicians can deny the seriousness of our situation. Indeed, the future of the human race is most clearly visible in our children. How threatened our future is becomes clear when contemplating just three instances among the many disturbing known facts:

- Since 1950, the human sperm count in the industrial world has gone down by 50%, primarily due to the sudden increase in pesticide use.[3]
- Over the last decade, cancer in children has increased by 200%, also primarily due to pesticide use.[4]
- Studies following several generations of children over two decades have shown that pregnant mothers exposed to low doses of pesticides give birth to children with irreversible and profound intellectual deficits.[5]

In 1996, Theo Colborn's **Our Stolen Future**[6] was published, with a foreword by then Vice-President Al Gore, providing the whole range of scientific evidence of this threat to human survival. In 1997, then US President Clinton issued an executive order in which he officially recognized the scientific basis for this threat and ordered as "a high priority" that pesticides and all endocrine-disrupting substances be identified and that all "environmental health risks affecting children" be assessed.[7] A long list of specifics followed, which resulted in all pesticides being brought under review, and some were taken out of circulation within months, others will no longer be produced, again others can only be used in low concentrations. Because of their different metabolisms, children are especially vulnerable to the effects of such toxins. In 2002, Canada's federal Health Minister incorporated the same protections for children in the new Pest Control Products Act. Many more initiatives, involving people at every stage of life, are underway throughout the world, among them environmental and orthomolecular medicine.

Environmental medicine treats those recently arisen illnesses caused by the contamination of air, water, and soil, and by food that is depleted of nutrients and contaminated by toxic additives. These new illnesses, such as Sick Building Syndrome and Multiple Chemical Sensitivity, have also come about through unhealthy workplaces and home environments. Well-known illnesses, such as cancer, asthma, diabetes and autoimmune disorders have increased to epidemic levels for the same reasons. The hallmark of environmentally mediated illness is that it appears at first totally mysterious, but almost always yields to a very simple explanation. It would be nice if one could add that these kinds of patients are a small minority. The fact is that, to a greater or lesser degree, this describes all of us.

Environmental medicine, like all good medicine, has an inescapable political component because that "very simple explanation" points always to the need for public action, political intervention, and the acknowledgement that we are almost always the authors of our own misfortunes. The history of public health measures supports this statement. Angry gods do not capriciously visit illness upon us. There is a rational explanation for human illness. We can understand the causes and we can respond intelligently to treat and prevent illness. How totally human health is dependent upon human behavior, nutritional choices, and anthropogenic environmental changes can be learned from the research in medical anthropology, which traces the origin and history of disease. This research has shown that this interdependent process can be traced back all the way into the paleolithic. Our current problems with cancer and chronic disease, caused by the sudden proliferation of toxic chemicals, is but the latest dramatic chapter in a long history.[8]

In the past, toxicology (which is an exact science like physics) was based on the dictum "the dose makes the poison," meaning that most substances an organism encountered were benign and became toxic only when reaching a critical strength. A tiny amount of poison, it was thought, was no problem; a large amount would kill you. Following the introduction of some 600,000 new synthetic chemicals since World War II, and the classic research by Rachel Carson[9] and other scientists, the principles of toxicology have fundamentally changed. We now know that frequent exposures to small amounts of toxins often have much more serious and deadly effects than a one-time big exposure. Tiny amounts of formaldehyde seeping into your home environment through insulation materials and furniture can ruin the lives of the entire family. The daily low-dose vapor of mercury coming from your "silver" amalgam tooth fillings can give you Alzheimer's disease years later.[10] A low-dose exposure to pesticides, or walking barefoot on pressure-treated wood during the critical early period of pregnancy, may cause your baby to be born with serious central nervous system defects.[5,11] These are just three examples. Therefore:

- *Environmental medicine is the clinical application of modern toxicology.*[12]
- *Environmental medicine is the clinical application of environmental biochemistry.*
- *Environmental doctors find the environmental sources of disease and develop non-toxic treatments and strategies for prevention.*
- *Environmental physicians use standard medical drugs whenever appropriate, but usually only as emergency measures because of the known toxicity of synthetic drugs; they favour biocompatible therapies, provide the patient with the knowledge of how to control the personal environment, cure the condition, or, at the very least, stabilize symptoms.*[13]
- *Environmental medicine works on solutions to general problems in medicine, such as antibiotic resistance and how to treat bacterial infections in patients who cannot tolerate antibiotics.*
- *Environmental medicine is not so much interested in categorizing a group of symptoms (i.e., a "diagnosis" for which a pharmaceutical agent is then usually targeted) as it is in assessing and correcting the numerous factors which have led an individual to feel pain, weakness, discomfort or disability, which are the definitions of illness, the reversal or alleviation of which is the goal of medicine.*
- *Because of its critical attitude, environmental medicine is especially interested in looking at well-known diseases such as arthritis, inflammatory bowel conditions, and autoimmune illnesses and often finds causes never before suspected—such as mycoplasma bacteria, which can cause classic lupus erythematosis, arthritis and scleroderma and are treatable by new, and often dramatically successful, protocols using standard antibiotics.*

- *Environmental medicine is also an international social movement, because physicians practicing it feel it is their inescapable responsibility to demand that the world should become once again fit for people to live in.*

ONE DOCTOR'S PRESCRIPTION FOR EVERY-DAY REBELLION

When you decide to take charge of your health, you stop functioning on automatic pilot. You no longer blindly trust your doctor because you suspect he or she can't know everything, either; you doubt the government's assurances on health matters because it is the nature of power to be in conflicts of interest; you question the advertisements on drugs because you realize that their aim is to sell drugs and not to cure you and thus lose a customer.[14] You listen to your body because it knows best; you are not a statistic or a population average, but a unique person with an individual genetic endowment and a very personal health history requiring personalized attention.[15] The health care industry, being as geared to mass production as the car industry, understandably finds that an inconvenience. Living things are characterized by diversity; even our sufferings are not created equal.

LIVING THINGS ARE CHARACTERIZED BY DIVERSITY; EVEN OUR SUFFERINGS ARE NOT CREATED EQUAL.

Without the birth of fundamental doubt and the growth of critical thinking, health is not possible, nor is advance in medicine. Doubt is the beginning of the cure. Trusting yourself is the first step on the road to recovery.[16] I would consider the effort of producing this book well worth it if it causes you to check for yourself the basis for the claims the health industry and doctors make (including myself!). That is why I hope this book will enable you to do two things for yourself and your loved ones:

1. *Learn that your environment causes or triggers specific health problems and what you can do to treat such problems and prevent them.*
2. *Have scientific and clinical ammunition with which to approach your doctors to help educate them.*

We need to know that human beings on planet earth are like fish in a tank of finite dimensions. As the Greek master physician, Hippocrates, taught 2,500 years ago, our health is determined by the air we breathe, the food we eat, the soil in which we grow it, the water we drink, and the way we feel and behave towards others. All illness and all health is ultimately a function of our physical and emotional environment. Even most genetically mediated illnesses are triggered by unhealthy environments and are ultimately preventable.

Second, modern medicine, ecology and biochemistry have provided us with the answers to the prevention of illness. Medical science has gone well beyond telling us not to smoke. We now know that we have to break the lethal dependence on toxic chemicals not only in ourselves, but also for our lawns, our agricultural practices, and our industrial economy. We can prevent cancer, heart disease, diabetes, arthritis, and many more illnesses. What's more, we can improve and very often even cure these illnesses. To foster your healthy doubt, I have provided an extensive bibliography, research and treatment resources, and even information on how doctors can obtain training in environmental medicine.

When you no longer blindly follow advice, but engage in a critical search for verifiable and workable solutions, you also begin the task of saving planet earth and human life. Like a stone thrown into a pool, the stone is small, but the ripples go on and on, covering immense distances for a very long time. In fact, what you actually do is to become politically engaged on behalf of life itself when you assume responsibility for what you eat and drink, what you permit to be in your surroundings, and what you will expose others to. You begin to make choices that have an effect on everything around you: your supermarket, your pharmacy, your local school, your garbage disposal, the way you furnish your home, the recreations you pursue, the car you buy, the information you spread among your friends and relatives.

WHEN YOU NO LONGER BLINDLY FOLLOW ADVICE, BUT ENGAGE IN A CRITICAL SEARCH FOR VERIFIABLE AND WORKABLE SOLUTIONS, YOU ALSO BEGIN THE TASK OF SAVING PLANET EARTH AND HUMAN LIFE.

Of course, you will always act on incomplete information (we all do, all of the time), but if you are in charge and engage your doctor in a critical dialogue and partnership, the result will always be better than whatever you got on automatic pilot.

The truth does make us free.

HOW I BECAME AN ENVIRONMENTAL PHYSICIAN

I was born in Poland and grew up on a farm. My family was poor, but we had enough to eat. As a child, I observed the brutalities of the Communist regime. Stalin's Soviet Union, which controlled Poland like a colony, ensured social "equality" in many cruel and absurd ways. When I was still a young boy, the "authorities" walked into our old farm house one day and removed everything we owned—not a stick of furniture was left, and they even took my mother's foot-treadle sewing machine, on which most of our clothes were made. The reasons for this action are as mysterious today as they were then. I can still remember the death of "Papa" Stalin in 1953. Loudspeakers in cars announced his death everywhere. The traffic stopped as if touched by a magic wand, and all pedestrians stood to attention, as did I. I was nine years old.

When I was fourteen, I contracted the Asiatic Flu and had a temperature of 40 degrees Celsius for several days. I recovered, but only temporarily, as the fever kept returning. The doctor assured my mother that I would be all right, but a mother's instinct often tends to be superior to a doctor's judgement, and she took me to a homeopath. He happened to be trained in iridology. He looked into my eyes and said, "There is something wrong with this boy's left lung." My mother took me at once to a tuberculosis hospital, where the diagnosis of pulmonary tuberculosis was confirmed. The recovery took the better part of a year, and during that time, I became very impressed with the doctors who took care of me. I promised myself that, if I recovered from this illness, I would become a doctor.

The ancient Greeks believed that the prerequisite for the practice of medicine was the experience of illness. The god of medicine, Asclepios, was known as the "wounded healer," because he had been struck by lightning and limped as a result. This prerequisite seems to hold true today especially for practitioners of environmental medicine. A medical journalist recently told me that a survey of the attending doctors at a recent *American Academy of Environmental Medicine* convention showed that most of them had themselves been seriously ill (or had a family member fall ill) with an environmentally-mediated condition for which their standard medical training had not prepared them.

In medical school, I soon discovered that nothing in life, least of all science, was free from the contamination of politics. University students were made to be part of the extensive spy system through which the Communist regimes supported their power. Students were expected to spy on their professors and report back to the Party on anything and everything "suspicious." To my horror, my favourite professor, who taught pediatrics, was assigned to me for surveillance when I became an assistant in pediatrics during my residency. The resulting emotional conflict was totally unbearable, and one day I decided I could not and would not do this, no matter what the consequences. I went straight to my professor and told him what I had been asked to do and that I would not do it. To my total surprise (and immeasurable relief), my professor smiled and said, "Oh, I know. I have known all along." That was the end of my involvement in the political spying business, and I somehow coasted through university politics in Communist Poland until 1972, when I completed my medical specialization in pediatrics —and escaped to Canada.

What precipitated this decision to escape was the following event. Early on in my pediatric training, in the early 1970s, I became interested in growth hormone research that had begun in the 1950s and which eventually led to its synthetic form. As I was a young pediatrician, the practical importance of this research for children whose growth is stunted, was clear. My first co-publications in peer-reviewed medical journals deal with growth hormone. I was in the university lab often seven days a week till the wee hours in the morning. One day I was working in the lab with a close friend of mine at about midnight, when we heard footsteps in the hall. To my speechless astonishment, my friend urged me to disappear as fast as possible into the men's room and stay there until he would come to fetch me. I did as he told me and waited, wondering what this could possibly be all about. After some time, he told me I could come out now. "What happened?" I asked. "Oh, I didn't want the head of the department to see you once again in the lab so late," he replied. Then I found out—and this was confirmed by others—that the department had become increasingly irritated with my enthusiasm for research. The word was out to "slow down Krop," as my performance was putting demands on the other department members that interfered with their more comfortable pace. Any serious hint of a desire for personal excellence was not encouraged in a collectivized society. That night, I knew I had to get out of Communist Poland.

In Canada, I needed to re-qualify. I was able to obtain an internship at Saskatoon City Hospital, where I worked from 1975 to 1976. By serendipity, I was assigned to Dr. Abram Hoffer for my rotation in psychiatry. Those three months totally transformed my approach to medicine. It was nothing less than a revolution for me. Here I saw people with severe psychiatric disorders being hospitalized and Dr. Hoffer—instead of prescribing tranquilizers and various psychotropic medication—gave them niacin (vitamin B_3), zinc and various other vitamins and minerals, as well as prescribing fundamental changes in their diets.[17] Their delusions disappeared, and they were returned to a normal life.

I could not believe it! Here I saw for the first time orthomolecular medicine in action—a branch of medicine I knew nothing about. All my training in Poland, then later at Sick Children's Hospital in Toronto, and in Saskatoon, up to this point, had been radically different and followed standard allopathic medicine. Dr. Hoffer also kept detailed patient charts. The descriptions of the patient's condition before and after treatment were very dramatic. His results were terrific, but he never pushed anything on his interns. It was simply through observation that one's eyes were opened to completely new possibilities in medicine. At the end of my internship with him, I asked him how I could learn more about orthomolecular medicine. "Well, if you are interested," he said in his typical low-key manner, "there are some books I would suggest." And so I began to read the work, among others, of Drs. H.L. Newbold, Carl C. Pfeiffer and Linus Pauling.[18]

After starting my own practice in 1977, I applied orthomolecular principles with great success for some time. However, I began to notice that some patients did not respond well enough. Vitamins, minerals and diet were simply not enough.

In 1979, one of my patients mentioned to me that there was a doctor in Hamilton, Ontario, who treated asthma successfully, not with steroids, but with sublingual desensitization drops. That was Dr. George John MacLennan. He was one of the founders of the Society for Clinical Ecology, now known as the *American Academy of Environmental Medicine* (AAEM), the study of which began with Dr. Theron Randolph of Chicago University in the 1940s.[19] Their observations and initial research laid a foundation through which environmental medicine spread throughout the world and became part of modern medical research. Dr. McLennan suggested that I attend the upcoming annual conference, which I did. At that conference, I was exposed to a new perspective on health and health problems and to the most generous and genuine physicians I had ever met. At that conference, I also saw a videotape of provocation-neutralization testing for food sensitivities done in Dr. Doris Rapp's medical office.[20]

Dr. Rapp was testing a child for food sensitivities, and when she tested for oats, the child had a dramatic reaction. This food actually had a neurotoxic effect and the child began to scream and thrash about. When Dr. Rapp finally established and administered the neutralizing dose, the child rapidly and totally recovered. Then Dr. Rapp asked the patient, "Do you remember anything that happened during the past two hours?" The child, genuinely bewildered, said, "No, I don't."

Well, at that point I got goosebumps and I knew, deep down and without any doubt, that this was the medicine I had to practice. Whatever I had learned in standard medicine did not even consider the neurotoxicity of ordinary foods—I had only been taught about IgE mediated allergies (regular hay fever and the like). What I had just seen was something completely different, and even if the biological pathways were not yet fully understood (as they are in the case of IgE-mediated allergies), here was the opportunity to understand and treat conditions otherwise simply discarded as "psychiatric"—unfair to psychiatry and brutally neglectful of the patient's real needs. The notion that such reactions could be treated with neutralizing doses of the offending substance, rather than with symptom-controlling drugs, was revolutionary. What's more, the same approach, I learned, could be taken in treating the toxic effects of environmental chemicals. The key point was that *the offending cause could be found, eliminated if possible and/or treated.* Standard medicine teaches how to classify symptoms, what drugs to use to control them, and how to use them cautiously to prevent their toxicity from killing the patient.

I went to Hamilton and took Dr. MacLennan's training course in environmental medicine. He also suggested I read a 700-page book by Lawrence Dickie entitled *Clinical Ecology* (C. Thomas Publications, Springfield, Ill. 1976). After reading about thirty pages of Dickie's book, I was overwhelmed and laid it aside and said to myself, "I won't be able to go through with this." I realized that I would be striking out in a 180-degree opposite direction to where all my colleagues were going. Dr. Theron Randolph used to warn young doctors, eager to learn the techniques of environmental medicine, saying ,"You realize this is a one-way street. There is no turning back." Not that the training I had had so far was useless—standard bacterial infection and trauma are perfectly treated by the standard medicine I had learned. However, chronic disease, which has become the subject of most of medicine, is dealt with primarily by symptom control, not finding causes and trying for a cure. I was devastated and actually rather scared.

It was clear to me that, if the findings and treatments of environmental and nutritional medicine would be taken seriously, the whole hefty bi-annually updated tome on internal medicine—the bible of the discipline—*Harrison's Principles of Internal Medicine*, would have to be fundamentally rewritten. Harrison's is like the huge descriptive treatises by the eighteenth and early ninteenth-century naturalists, who classified and described the natural world in every minute detail without being able to explain any of that diversity and how it all hangs together, until Charles Darwin in 1859 provided a dynamic explanation for evolution, and modern genetics proved that it all does hang together as one huge web of life.

It was an intense— but not a very long—war that I waged within myself. It was the patients that decided it in the end. Whenever I looked at them with the search frame of standard medicine, and then again with that of environmental medicine, I quickly knew what I had to do. The patient's environmental exposure and nutritional history generally explained the causes of the observed signs and symptoms often quite elegantly and rationally. Symptom-control became intolerably frustrating. So, I returned to the study of Dickie's book and took every available course, including one intense one with Dr. Theron Randolph himself. I am still taking courses every year. The treatment protocols environmental physicians use are regularly adjusted to take advantage of new research and information. Unfortunately, however, there are powerful forces opposing this progress.

THE HAZARDS OF BEING AN ENVIRONMENTAL PHYSICIAN

Not only do we have to detoxify on a daily basis the carcinogenic and hormone-disrupting chemicals and synthetic materials we ingest through water, air, and food—we also have to deal with the dead weight of outdated and intellectually toxic ideas which make the birth of the new always so difficult and even outright prevent good medicine from reaching patients. I knew from my teachers in environmental medicine that doing medicine in this new and revolutionary manner could be dangerous to one's professional health. After all, identifying pesticides, petrochemicals, many symptom-controlling drugs, and processed foods (to name just a few serious health hazards) as the causes of cancer and chronic diseases is not going to make a doctor very popular with the captains of industry. The findings of environmental medicine, and the demonstration that avoiding all these toxic substances can restore people's health, constitute a most formidable critique of our modern world and its commercial values.

Medical regulatory bodies today are slow to tolerate new approaches, not only because bureaucracies have always been slow to accept any sort of progress, but because the values dominant in a bureaucracy are far removed from the values that guide a doctor in his real-life relationship to the patient. Medical regulatory bodies are as conflicted in their interests as they were 150 years ago, when bacteria were the heresy of the day and washing one's hands, before examining a patient or performing surgery, was an affront to professional pride. Finally, while ethics demands that medicine should be free of commercial interests, the fact is that symptom control is a multi-billion dollar business and not likely to take the back seat without a fight. Symptom control is the market, and wealth is measured in this market, as in any other, by growth, not by the diminishing returns cures would generate.

Indeed, we have become so used to the priority of all commercial concerns—to the rights of every "stakeholder," with the patient being merely the consumer—that we have effectively ceased to even question something as ethically incomprehensible as the following fact: the very councils of Canada's Colleges of Physicians and Surgeons, which control medical practice and standards, have on them non-elected, appointed members who directly come from, or are associated with, the pharmaceutical and insurance industries. Those non-medical members are even permitted to sit on disciplinary committees. Even the *elected* members have their research funded by those same companies—nobody is free. The standard of medicine is determined by forces that have little to do with curing sick people.[21]

As for the practicing doctor, the fact also is that most learn new information primarily from the drug company representatives who visit their offices regularly (see endnote 14). An astonishing 80% of all Canadian physicians have some financial tie to the pharmaceutical industry (*Globe & Mail*,

Feb. 6, 2002), which a recent editorial in the *Journal of the Canadian Medical Association* described as a relationship akin to "dancing with the porcupine."[22]

One Canadian doctor published the total number of visits and personalized mailings he received from drug companies in *The Medical Post* (Feb. 9, 1999): the total was 452 promotional encounters in one year.

ONE CANADIAN DOCTOR PUBLISHED THE TOTAL NUMBER OF VISITS AND PERSONALIZED MAILINGS HE RECEIVED FROM DRUG COMPANIES IN THE *MEDICAL POST* (FEB. 9, 1999): THE TOTAL WAS 452 PROMOTIONAL ENCOUNTERS IN ONE YEAR.

As for medical research, it is hardly surprising that research capable of generating patentable high-tech treatments, promising the dependence of large numbers of people, gets the grant money, almost all of which comes from the pharmaceutical companies. (In continental Europe, most research is paid for by governments and, therefore, truly independent and not so drug-oriented.) Following the recent revelations about how Dr. Nancy Olivieri[23] was ordered by a drug company to remain silent about the dangers of one of their drugs she was researching, *Doctors for Research Integrity* was created to protect researchers from drug companies' commercial priorities. Indeed, the concept of "research integrity" is in danger of becoming as much an oxymoron at Canada's "health protection branch." Drs. Shiv Chopra and Margaret Haydon had to take the Canadian government to court in order to establish their right and scientific duty to warn the Canadian public of the dangers to their food supply from unlawfully introduced carcinogens and hormone disrupting chemicals. They won that precedent-setting case in a federal court decision in 2000.[24]

The environmental physician is also pitted against much government policy on a national and international level. Speaking the truth about what we see in our patients on a daily basis—carcinogens and neurotoxins in their blood, pesticides in their fat biopsies, heavy metals in their urine and stools—is nothing less than a total indictment of governments that have ceased to be regulators and protectors of society and become publicly funded butlers serving the big corporations.

The history of medicine is full of martyrs, and I had no intention of joining their ranks. In fact, I am cursed with an enthusiasm for stuff that works, and I became entangled in the politics of medicine despite my best efforts to stay out of politics! When scientific paradigms clash, it is much like a tectonic shift: one gets caught in a huge social upheaval and does one's best to defend the facts and basic principles. And so I fought a thirteen-year battle with the College of Physicians and Surgeons of Ontario (CPSO), the body that licenses doctors in this province. This disciplinary ordeal was not based on patient complaints—on the contrary, my trial was energetically opposed by my patients, my colleagues, the general public, and even politicians.

Th CPSO *formally charged* me with suggesting to patients they drink uncontaminated water, have air filters installed to alleviate asthma, eat organically grown foods free of carcinogenic pesticides, utilize detoxification protocols for solvents and pesticides, etc. The treatments used by environmental doctors, such as the provocation-neutralization technique described above, the various detoxification and diet-centered therapies, the use of vitamins and minerals as therapies, and the diagnoses of illnesses such as Multiple Chemical Sensitivity, Sick Building Syndrome and Candidiasis—all were *formulated as charges*, and I was, after a four-year trial, found "guilty" of their use. The entire body of scientific evidence from the world's leading medical journals and the World Health Organization, which I provided through my lawyers, was rejected, as were my defence witnesses, even though they came from Johns Hopkins Medical School, the medical schools of the Universities of Toronto, Saskatchewan, Nova Scotia, Stanford, and from the various government-sponsored environmental health clinics of Canada, the US and Europe. I am now asking the Supreme Court of Canada for leave to appeal the absurdity of having an entire branch of medicine arbitrarily condemned.

All this took place in spite of the fact that the patient charts showed that patients had greatly benefited from these treatments—a fact even the CPSO tribunal acknowledged in their decision! Most of the very patients whose charts had been used to formulate the charges protested and testified on my behalf at the end of the trial. The purpose of this trial—possibly the longest disciplinary investigation in medical history—was made very clear in the official Sentence handed down by the CPSO in 1999:

1. *"Dr. Krop must make it clear to his patients that the diagnoses and therapies…are unsupported by scientifically acceptable evidence."*
2. *"Members of the profession at large—a profession whose integrity rests on the practice of scientifically based medicine—must know why and how Dr. Krop's practice fails the standard."*
3. *"The public…must be protected from practitioners who lack that credibility."*

The motives for rejecting all of the defence's scientific evidence supporting environmental medicine's treatment and diagnostic modalities can only be guessed at. Just how far out of touch with medical reality the CPSO Decision is becomes clear when considering the following:

The United Nations Environment Programme issued its GEO-3 Report, to which more than a thousand scientists contributed (*Nature*, May 30th, 2002, p. 475). It states that "the benefits of some environmentally friendly policies will not be apparent until decades after they have been enacted." The report states that "even if environmentally friendly approaches were adopted now, carbon dioxide concentrations would continue to rise until 2050. Water shortages would continue and coastal pollution would increase slightly." The cartoon that went with it showed a speedboat named "Human Behavior" cruising full speed ahead towards the edge of an abyss. Its pilot, a skeleton, said with his head turned to the terrified passengers, "Brakes? What brakes?"

I wrote this primer to enable you to find out what environmental medicine can do for you and to introduce you to the excellent science on which these therapies are based. I have also provided in its appendix the treatment protocols for some of the most serious environmentally-mediated conditions. They are intended for you to research and to use for the purpose of making an informed decision. In medicine, everything ultimately originates in patient experience, so you need to judge for yourself how much of what you read applies to you and how much does not.

MEDICINE, THE HOUSE OF MANY MANSIONS

Paraphrasing the saying by Jesus, "In my father's house are many mansions," it is vital to understand that there are many ways by which an illness can be cured, and new approaches are being discovered and will continue to be developed. Only fools and those with a vested interest believe they control and have the one and only answer.

I was trained in twentieth-century medicine, and it is my conviction that the focus of environmental medicine is the natural evolution of medical science at its best. Environmental medicine developed in response to the devastation of our planetary life-support systems, just as bacteriological medicine developed as a response to the objective findings that bacteria and dirt can cause disease. Both these advances were stimulated by the tremendous breakthroughs in technology which enabled scientists and doctors to see what was previously mysterious. Similarly, the possibilities now open to doctors with regard to early detection of pathology, the analyses of a person's biological material enabling one to see what is happening on the cellular level—all this is a fabulous tool bag the previous generation of physicians merely dreamed of as science fiction. As a physician, I am amazed by and grateful for the use of all of these diagnostic and therapeutic modalities.

Environmental medicine depends upon and arises out of the discoveries being made in endocrinology, immunology, biochemistry and cell biology as much as it does on the research results in all the ecological sciences, toxicology, and especially epidemiology. All of life is interdependent in sickness and in health. Environmental medicine differs from traditional medicine only in that it can—in the face of the overwhelming evidence—no longer look at patients and their presenting pathology and complaints isolated from the air, water, soil, food, workplace, home environment, and emotional life of that person's environment. Environmental medicine broadens the perspective of medicine as a whole. It vastly increases our understanding of everything in medicine and increases our options dramatically. Consider how the various medical specialities can benefit and improve patient outcome by adding these new insights to all that is already known and found to be beneficial through long experience:

- *The surgeon can have better results in wound healing if the knowledge of vitamins and other vital nutrients is incorporated in the treatment of trauma;[25] long-term problems are prevented by ensuring that the intravenous delivery system (tubes, bags, etc.) do not contain endocrine-disrupting phthalates (now beginning to be phased out in hospitals).*

- *The pediatrician treating childhood asthma need no longer worry about the long-term detrimental effects of steroid inhalers when it is so often possible to eliminate the cause, such as food intolerance or toxic chemicals in the home or school environment.[26]*

- *The gerontologist can help restore a considerable measure of independence to many Alzheimer's patient by eliminating the causal dental mercury amalgam and by chelating a lifetime's stored body burden of toxic metals.[27]*

- *The urologist, frustrated by the lack of success with antibiotics in patients plagued by recurrent cystitis and urinary tract infections, can cure most of these patients by dealing with the generally underlying candidiasis or e-coli infection through the use of probiotics, various friendly bacteria and dietary adjustments.[28]*

- *The rheumatologist can expand treatment options dramatically by looking for mycoplasma as the cause in many cases of arthritis and scleroderma, both of which will respond to the old standby—antibiotics used in new treatment protocols; alternatively, many arthritis patients respond well to the elimination of certain foods they are unknowingly sensitive to, such as coffee and the deadly nightshade family of plants (potatoes, tomatoes, peppers etc.)[29]*

- *The neurologist, usually helpless when facing terrible diseases such as multiple sclerosis, myasthenia gravis, or Parkinson's, can with environmental toxins in mind turn to detoxification and subsequent restorative nutrient enhancement protocols that often not only arrest the progress of these diseases, but actually can cure them.[30]*

- *The gynecologist familiar with natural hormone therapy can treat everything from endometriosis to menopause and not be concerned about potential deadly side effects in the long run. The revelations about the carcinogicity of synthetic hormones, currently dominating the news, are nothing new to the environmentally trained physician: we have known this for at least two decades and have avoided their use in our patients.[31]*

- *For the oncologist, the tedious writing of death certificates is beginning to give way to a whole new world of healing and prevention opened up by orthomolecular and nutritional medicine as their success, with even the most virulent cancers, achieved by the Gerson Institute, the work of Dr. Nicholas Gonzales and other researchers in this area is now finally being taken seriously by medical research.[32]*

- *The physician treating heart cardiovascular disease can more often than not avoid bypass surgery through chelation therapy, dietary and lifestyle adjustments and the dramatic healing effects of vitamin E and niacin, as well as other nutrients. (This treatment is now protected by law in Alberta since 1997.) (See endnote 27)*

- *The psychiatrist, as I learned from Dr. Abraham Hoffer in the early 1970s, can offer control over some of the most debilitating mental conditions with the new knowledge nutritional biochemistry has made available about the role of essential fatty acids, minerals and vitamins (e.g., niacin) and herbal medicines (e.g., St. John's Wort) in mental disease.[33]*

All this information comes from the world's most prestigious medical research institutions and is found in the international medical journals available to all doctors (and patients) through the Internet search engines that access medical libraries.

As for drugs, used appropriately and in pharmacological doses, they are most certainly at times miraculous and indispensable. I certainly use antibiotics, drugs that control fungi and parasites, various steroids and hormones and pain medication in my practice. The art of medicine, however, is to help the patient back to a normal, productive life, such that the person is hopefully no longer dependent on the doctor or on any drugs! Used long-term, and without regard for the bioindividuality of the patient, modern drugs can be deadly. In 1998, the University of Toronto and the American FDA published the results of a large meta-analysis which showed that the side effects of *properly prescribed drugs taken as prescribed* are the fourth leading cause of death in North America.[34] Dr. Jay Cohen, a professor of preventive medicine at the University of California in San Diego, published an astounding book, *Overdose*. His survey of the medical literature shows— and his own clinical experience confirmed—that just about every drug is basically overdose and hence dangerous and even lethal. In fact, the rate of death from apparently properly prescribed medication would, according to his research, be much higher than previously thought (see endnote 35). The reason is, he writes, that the drug companies create one-size-fits-all drugs to make them easier to market and inflate effectiveness statistics. Coming from the orthodox medical community, this is a very serious condemnation indeed.[35]

What sets environmentally trained doctors apart is the way we take a patient history, because we see human beings embedded in the whole of Nature. When we take a history, we listen, and listen, and listen, and listen— and visualize our patient in their personal environment. No detail is too trivial and will include the carpeting, the method of heating, the location of the garage, the possible fungi in the bathroom, the foods most frequently eaten, a recent change of location, the air-conditioning, the windows (or lack thereof) in the office, the brand of shampoo, etc., and our questionnaires are very long—exhaustive and exhausting!

As I stated before the Brundtland Commission, medicine needs to get out of the eighteenth-century philosophy that sees the body as a machine, the paradigm that caused medical science to split into specialties and sub-specialties such that nothing hangs together anymore. A machine is not dependent upon Nature. Hippocrates taught us about the effects of food, occupation, and the quality of water and air, on health. His book entitled *Air, Water and Places* provided 2,500 years ago the basic concepts of what today we call ecology. That extreme specialization has brought much knowledge, to be sure; but organisms are dynamic functioning totalities, not parts. When something goes wrong, always the totality is affected. A headache can ruin your day completely, even though the rest of your body works fine. Cancer, no matter where it is located, is a systemic disease, not a partial malfunction.

The word "doctor" comes from the Latin "docere," meaning "to teach." Teaching health should once again be central to the job description of every physician. It is important, but not sufficient, to tell people to stop smoking, eat more vegetables and take more exercise. What is the point of eating more vegetables if they are loaded with carcinogenic pesticides? It is the aim of every environmental doctor to equip patients with knowledge they can use to make their own homes, gardens and workplaces supportive of life and teach their family, friends and employers what can be done to prevent illness.

CAUSE FOR CAUTIOUS OPTIMISM

As doctors and patients, we have our work cut out for us. Health has become the number one political and economic issue worldwide. Currently, in Canada, the Romanow Commission is understandably primarily concerned about how to make universal health care work when its cost is out of control. It is, therefore, extremely important to understand that an environmentally oriented approach to medicine is infinitely cheaper than the high-tech symptom-control approach so popular in standard medicine, primarily because it does not need patentable therapies to achieve results.

- *In 1981, the prestigious mainstream medical journal,* **Annals of Allergy,** *published the results of a five-year follow-up on two sets of patients suffering from thrombophlebitis. There were ten patients in each group. The group treated by conventional methods had more than two hundred* *flare-ups during that five-year period. The group treated by environmental medicine methods (nutrition, vitamins etc.) only reported two flare-ups. The first group had a total of 114 hospitalizations to report, while those treated according to environmental medicine techniques did not have a single hospitalization to report. Only one of the conventionally treated patients was able to return to work, while all ten of the other group returned to work. Costs for the conventional group was a total of US $300,000 during that period, while the environmental medicine patients spent a total of US $2,500.[36]*

- *In 1998, the German government published the results of a government-funded pilot project: a hospital specializing in environmental medicine, located in Bredsted. The results were so impressive, the German government decided to build four more such hospitals.[37]*

- *I take comfort in the fact that over the past decade, virtually every university in the industrialized world has begun to offer some courses in environmentally oriented medicine.*

- *The agricultural departments of the European Union, led by Denmark, have made organic agriculture their top priority.*

- *The international POP's Treaty (on persistent organic pesticides) was ratified.*

- *The US National Institutes of Health is funding the research into Dr. Nicholas Gonzales' successful alternative cancer therapy.*

- *Through the American Association for the Advancement of Science and the US National Center for Environmental Health, the US government in 2000 started an ambitious program of testing thousands of people annually for all the various toxic substances in their blood and establishing a government registry to trace their sources and effects—a fundamental necessity if we are ever to clean up the human organism. (According to Johns Hopkins Medical School, of the 3,000 most frequently used chemicals, only 7% have safety screening data.)*

- *In the UK, the House of Lords commissioned major research into pesticides and has taken a proactive stance in protective legislation.*

- *Following the recent "Hudson Decision" by the Canadian Supreme Court, city after city is banning the use of pesticides and pressure-treated wood in Canada. Similar efforts have begun in the US.*
- *I already mentioned the successful efforts by scientists such as Drs. Chopra, Haydon and Olivieri. Due to their determined refusal to bow to vested interests and political pressure, dangerous drugs are being kept from entering our food supply. Bovine growth hormone (a known carcinogen and endocrine disrupter) was not only forbidden in Canada due to Drs. Chopra and Haydon's efforts at Health Canada, but the facts about BGH thus became available to the European Union, where this synthetic hormone was also banned. Furthermore, Dr. Olivieri has taken up the battle against unsafe drugs with court action in the European Union as well.*
- *The national medical associations of North America and Europe not only give full study credits for doctors pursuing environmental medicine education, but are working on new guidelines to get control over the rampant conflict of interest in medical research.*
- *Thanks to the efforts of Dr. Lynn Marshall at the Environmental Health Clinic at Women's College Hospital in Toronto, the Canadian Medical Association Journal recently published a six-part series on environmental medicine, introducing doctors to its protocols and diagnoses.[38]*
- *It is a pleasure to recall that Canada led the way for North America in focusing on the seriousness of the environmentally mediated health problems, first through the Thomson Commission in 1985 (for which my practice was chosen to serve as a major source of information), and then through a series of workshops, symposia and research projects funded by Health Canada and the universities of Toronto and Dalhousie.[39]*
- *Most heartening is the voluntary initiative to clean up this polluted earth coming from industry. David Suzuki, in his latest book,* Good News for a Change: Hope for a Troubled Planet *(David Suzuki; Holly Dressel, Stoddart, 2002) describes these developments.*

I am personally encouraged by the increasing number of "pesky" patients everywhere! Most of my patients have slogged, on average, through at least seven doctors' offices (the last one was usually a psychiatrist) and persevered until they were finally taken seriously. I was amused to learn that in June 2002 the same observation was troubling the delegates attending the international convention of medical regulatory agencies, hosted by my very own CPSO. They agreed that patients today no longer just accept what they are told. They come to their doctors having researched their health problems and wish to engage their physicians in discussion. One of the speakers from the UK lamented that control is just not what it used to be. Thank God for that!

Most amazing of all, I never cease to be astonished by the resilience of the human body—Nature's stubborn urge to heal that cooperates with the doctor's efforts and keeps the patient going with tireless patience. Nature's determination to restore what is injured is the constant source of hope and courage for patient and doctor.

Jozef J. Krop
Mississauga, Ontario, August 2002

ENDNOTES

1 WORLD COMMISSION ON ENVIRONMENT AND DEVELOPMENT, Our Common Future, Oxford, 1987

2 My submission was later published in *Clinical Ecology*, Vol. IV, No.3, 1986

3 Web site for the World Health Organization: **http://www.who.int/en/**

4 Statistics presented at McMaster University, Hamilton, Ontario, Canada, 1999, by Dr. S. Epstein at *Everyday Carcinogens: Stopping Cancer Before it Starts*, transcripts available through Canadian Environmental Law Association, Suite 401, 517 College Street, Toronto, ON, M6G 4A2, or download from **www.stopcancer.org**.

5 For pesticides and fetal development: S. STEINGRABER, Having Faith, Perseus, Cambridge Mass., 2001.

6 T. COLBORN et al, *Our Stolen Future*, Plume-Penguin, New York, 1997

7 The text of this presidential order of April 21, 1997, can be downloaded from the US government site: **www.health.gov/environment/TaskForce/whouseprenv.html**

8 M.N. COHEN, *Health and the Rise of Civilization*, Yale University Press, 1989

9 R. CARSON, *Silent Spring*, (1962), Houghton Mifflin, Co., New York, 25th anniversary edition, 1987

10 S. KHATOON et al. "Aberrant Guanosine Triphosphate-Beta-Tubulin Interaction in Alzheimer's Disease" in *Annals of Neurology*, vol. 26, no. 2, 1989. The most comprehensive source for primary research and clinical applications in this area is the *International Academy for Oral and Medical Toxicology* at **www.IAOMT.org** or Tel: (863) 420-6373

11 For pressure-treated wood hazards: **http://www.noccawood.ca/** or e-mail: **deborahbarrie@hotmail.com**

12 T. G. RANDOLPH, M.D., *Human Ecology and Susceptibility to the Chemical Environment*, 7th printing, Charles C. Thomas, Springfield, Ill., 1980. The most comprehensive treatment of the subject is the 4-volume work by W. J. RAE, M.D., *Chemical Sensitivity*, Volumes 1–4, Lewis Publishers, 1992-1996

13 According to the *Journal of the American Pharmaceutical Association* 41:192-99, 2001, for every US $1.11 spent on a prescription drug, another US $1.77 needs to be spent to treat the harmful side effects of that drug.

14 J. ROBINSON, *Prescription Games*, McClelland & Stewart Ltd., Toronto, 2001

15 R. J. WILLIAMS, *Biochemical Individuality*, (1956), Keats, New Canaan, Ct., 1998

16 One of my colleagues observed, in summing up a lecture comparing the poor outcomes of standard cancer treatment (chemotherapy and radiation) with the excellent results obtained by using vitamins, minerals, amino-acids, enzymes, specialized diets, and detoxification protocols: "… and so the results show that if you take conventional treatment, you die a conventional death." Dr. Michael Gonzales at the *30th Annual International Conference*, Toronto, May 2001

[17] A. HOFFER, M.D., *Vitamin B-3 & Schizophrenia: Discovery, Recovery, Controversy*, Quarry Health Books, Kingston, ON, Canada, 1998 (this is the new and updated edition of the research published in the 1950s–1970s). A comprehensive overview of orthomolecular medicine, also for patients is in A. HOFFER, *Orthomolecular Medicine for Physicians*, Keats, New Canaan, Ct., 1989

[18] The many publications by Linus Pauling and complete access to the worldwide research on vitamins and orthomolecular medicine is available through the *Linus Pauling Institute* at Oregon State University, 571 Weniger Hall, Corvallis, Oregon, 97331-6512, or **http://lpi.oregonstate.edu/**.

[19] T. RANDOLPH, M.D., *Environmental Medicine: Beginnings & Bibliographies of Clinical Ecology*, Clinical Ecology Publications Inc., Fort Collins, CO, 1987

[20] D. RAPP, M.D., *Is This Your Child?*, Quill-William Morrow, New York, 1991. The video tapes of Dr. Rapp's clinical work and other information for parents can be obtained from: *Practical Allergy Research Foundation*, P.O. Box 60, Buffalo, New York, 14223-0060. The classic in this field is T. RANDOLPH, M.D., *An Alternative Approach to Allergies*, Revised Edition, Harper & Row, New York, 1990

[21] An affidavit filed by my defence lawyers on December 3, 1995, with the CPSO disciplinary tribunal, outlined how the expert witnesses, whom the prosecution was going to call, were compromised by conflicts of interest. For example, the 16-page affidavit stated with regard to two of these witnesses: "Drs. S. and M. have a personal stake in the outcome of the Disciplinary Committee's decision by reason of their financial ties to those drug companies whose interest lies in opposition to Dr. Krop. Dr.M. has, from 1985 to 1995, received over one million, three hundred thousand dollars in grants from drug manufacturers Sandoz, Upjohn, Fisons, Schering, Astra, Ciba-Geigy, Janssen Glaxo and Abbott." The reason this situation represented a conflict of interest was because the drugs researched by these prosecution witnesses were of the kind that the treatment modalities of environmental medicine render unnecessary. These treatment modalities were what I was defending.

[22] CMAJ editorial, Sept. 18, 2001

[23] J. THOMPSON et al, *The Olivieri Report*, Canadian Association of University Teachers, 2001

[24] On the Internet, you will find more than 400 references and informational items about the efforts of Dr. Shiv Chopra and his colleagues at Health Canada to inform the public about the dangers posed to our food supply by carcinogens and endocrine disrupters. Search under "Shiv-Chopra."

[25] A.DAVIS, *Let's Get Well*, Signet, New York, 1972

[26] R. FIRSHEIN, *Reversing Asthma*, Warner Books, New York, 1998.

[27] M. WALKER, et al. *The Chelation Answer*, Second Opinion Publishing, Atlanta, Georgia, 1994. As chelation is an excellent therapy also for diabetic neuropathy, heart and cardio-vascular disease, good sources of information are the ALTERNATIVE MEDICINE GUIDE volume *Heart Disease, Stroke & High Blood Pressure* by the Burton Goldberg Group, Future Medicine Publishing, 1998 and cardiothoracic surgeon M. OZ's *Healing from the Heart*, Plume Books, New York, 1998.

28 ALTERNATIVE MEDICINE GUIDE, *Women's Health Series* vol. 1, Burton Goldberg Group, Future Medicine Publishing, New York, 1998. W.G. CROOK, M.D., *The Yeast Connection Handbook*, Professional Books Inc., Jackson, Tennessee, 1998

29 Alternative Medicine Guide, *Arthritis*, Burton Goldberg Group, Alternative Medicine Books, 1999. J.B. IRWIN, M.D., *Arthritis Be Gone!*, Keats Publishing, New Canaan, Ct., 1997. S.A. ROGERS, M.D., *Pain Free in Six Weeks*, Sandkeye Co. Sarasota, FL., 2001

30 The Klenner Protocol (after Dr. F.R. Klenner) for Multiple Sclerosis and Myasthenia gravis was originally published in the *Journal of Applied Nutrition* in 1973 and is available through The Towensend Letter for Doctors and Patients at 360-385-6021 or http://www.tldp.com

31 U. REISS, M.D., *Natural Hormone Balance for Women*, Pocket Books New York, 2001. D.L. BERKSON, *Hormone Deception*, Contemporary Books, New York, 2000

32 The research papers and treatment information by Dr. N. GONZALES can be downloaded from his web site at **www.dr-gonzalez.com**. The currently ongoing research at the National Institutes of health into the Gonzales treatment can be downloaded for free from the web site of the US National Cancer Institute at **www.cancer.gov**

33 M. PEET, I. GLEN, D.F. HORROBIN, *Phospholipid Spectrum Disorder in Psychiatry*, Marius Press, UK, 199:, contains the medical scientific research for the specialist. For the general reader are recommended: A. HOFFER, M.D., *Putting It All Together: The New Orthomolecular Nutrition*, Keats, New Canaan, CT., 1996

34 J. LAZAROU, B.H. POMERANZ, P.N. COREY, "Incidence of Adverse Drug Reactions in Hospitalized Patients," Journal of the American Medical Association, April 15, 1998, vol. 279, no. 15. For an overview on specific dangerous drugs see CBC Ideas, transcript of "Naked in the Pharmaceutical Marketplace," 2001, **http://www.cbc.ca/ideas/**

35 J.S. COHEN, M.D., *Overdose: The Case Against the Drug Companies*, Tarcher-Putnam, New York, 2001

36 W.J. RAE et al. "Recurrent environmentally triggered thrombophlebitis: a five-year followup." *Annals of Allergy* 47:338-44, 1981

37 The German Government's report on the Bredstedt environmental medicine clinic is entitled *Abschlussbericht: Umweltmedizinische Ambulanz Bredstedt*, published by the University of Luebeck, available through Institut fur Sozialmedizin, Beckergrube 43-47, 23552 Luebeck, Germany

38 *Canadian Medical Association Journal* series on environmental medicine is published in vol. 166, no. 8 (April 16, 2002), no. 9 (April 30), no. 10 (May 14), no. 11 (May 28), no. 12 (June 11), no. 13 (June 25)

39 See historical overview regarding the impact of the 1985 Thomson Report to the Ontario Ministry of Health in N. ASHFORD & C. MILLER, *Chemical Exposure: Low Levels and High Stakes*, second edition, Van Nostrand Reinhold, 1998

Principles of Environmental Medicine

PRINCIPLES

To understand any illness, we must look at the environmental aspects of health and disease. Centuries ago, the Greek philosopher and physician, Aristotle, taught, "to understand the man one has to understand the environment he lives in." His disciple, Hippocrates, carried on this philosophy in his teaching and his work. In his book, *Air, Water and Places*, he developed the practical application of this concept, looking at how air, water, soil and food have an effect on health and disease of human beings. Environmental medicine combines those basic principles, with modern diagnostic techniques to treat many immune related diseases.

In today's world, many illnesses are the result of reactions to substances found in the places where we live, work, and go to school. Many chronic illnesses, such as autoimmune disorders, including lupus erythematosus, juvenile onset diabetes mellitus, rheumatoid arthritis, and multiple sclerosis, can be triggered by environmental factors, particularly toxic chemicals. Patients with environmental illness usually present with multisystemic disorders,

> MANY CHRONIC ILLNESSES, SUCH AS AUTOIMMUNE DISORDERS, INCLUDING LUPUS ERYTHEMATOSUS, JUVENILE ONSET DIABETES MELLITUS, RHEUMATOID ARTHRITIS, AND MULTIPLE SCLEROSIS, CAN BE TRIGGERED BY ENVIRONMENTAL FACTORS, PARTICULARLY TOXIC CHEMICALS.

including the central nervous system, which is particularly sensitive to toxins. The symptoms can usually be traced to specific causative factors found in surrounding environmental exposures, diet or drugs.

Our body is built from elements of the external environment, arranged according to the genetic coding of the Deoxyribonucleic acid (DNA), which we received from our parents. These elements are supplied through the foods we eat. It is important to realize that during our cultural evolution we have continually contaminated the environment, and at the same time introduced an overabundance of non-nutritious "junk foods." With the introduction of toxins and extensive agricultural techniques, the soil, the base of the food chain, has become deficient in many basic nutrients (i.e., magnesium, zinc, vitamins, etc.). As a result, foods produced contain too many toxic substances and are deficient in some nutrients. *Poor availability of appropriate nutrients for the human body has a negative effect not only on its structure but also on its function.* There are two important aspects in this area: genetic makeup of generations to come and poor functioning of the central nervous system.

Genetic information contained in the DNA is basically identical today to the information contained thousands of years ago. This information dictates how to build, as well as how to regenerate our bodies. Since the quality of our daily food intake has decreased, it is not comparable to the parameters coded in the DNA. This means that the human organism builds and regenerates itself from poor quality materials. *By analogy, it could be compared to building a home according to sound architectural plans, but using substandard materials. The end result will be a house that looks exactly as planned by the architect (DNA), but will be more vulnerable to destruction.* It would seem that the contemporary human body is in a parallel situation.

One of my mentors, Prof. Dr. Julian Aleksandrowicz of Krakow, shared the following thoughts with me: A human being is only able to maintain his or her integrity, identity and sovereignty as long as the psychological processes are energetically supported by the correct supply of nutrients and oxygen. Intoxicated brain function becomes subclinically abnormal: When the battery of a calculator begins to weaken, the calculator can perform only simple functions and fails with complicated ones. A polluted brain works, by analogy, in the same way. It can perform its basic functions (brain stem functions) of maintaining breathing, circulation, instincts of sex and hunger, but higher functions (cortical) such as learning, love, friendship, sharing and social responsibility become distorted. Maintenance of body structure and function can only be achieved through sustainable management of our environment.

Furthermore, neurobehavioral toxicology proves that toxins, even in a very small dose, can change the human brain, and more so, the very vulnerable brains of developing children. These toxins can cause decreased intellectual functioning and even hallucination.

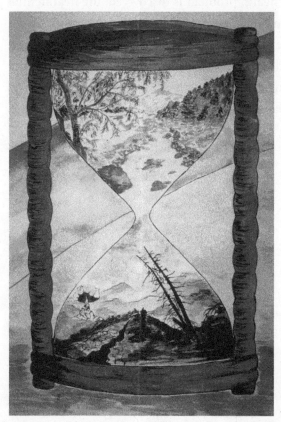

Polish Ecological Club:
Ecological Poster Contest for
Youth, Earth Day 1991.
Artist: Iwona Brojewska

WHAT IS ENVIRONMENTAL MEDICINE?

Environmental medicine provides a real understanding of any disease process by taking into consideration an individual's genetic endowment, as well as environmental stressors (immediate, local and global). Ironically it is very closely related to the original thoughts and teachings of Hippocrates, which had mostly been forgotten until recently.

Environmental Medicine (EM), or Clinical Ecology as it is also referred to, is the medical discipline which studies and assesses the effect of environmental factors upon individuals with particular emphasis on the effect of foods, chemicals, water, indoor and outdoor air quality, at home, work or school. It considers each patient as an exceptional individual exposed to a unique set of circumstances and needing a custom-tailored therapy.

Once the cause of the health problem is discovered, the treatment is as direct as possible with minimal use of pharmaceutical drugs, effectively avoiding any adverse side effects. Treatment consists of environmental controls, diet modification, nutritional supplements and immunotherapy (injectable and/or sublingual), detoxification (I.V., sauna), modification of metabolic/hormonal imbalances with natural products/hormones, chelation for heavy metals, cardiovascular and degenerative disorders etc.

The father of Environmental Medicine, Theron G. Randolph, originally designed this logo. It encompasses the interrelationship between Adaptation, Allergy, Nutrition and Toxicology as it pertains to the practice and understanding of Environmental Medicine.

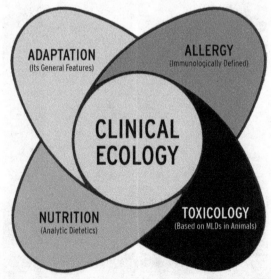

Environmental   vs.   Allopathic Medicine

HISTORY

- Reviews symptoms involving each system and searches for environmental contributors to illness.
- History of dietary and environmental factors are considered in arriving at a diagnosis.

- Takes history relating only to organ-oriented problems for different specialties, e.g., neurology, nephrology, cardiology, etc., with a limited emphasis on dietary habits and minimal attention to environmental factors.

STAGE OF DISEASE

- Diagnosis can be made in subclinical, pre-morbid state before end-organ damage.

- End-organ damage must be present to diagnose and treat.

FOCUS OF MEDICAL ATTENTION

- Focus is holistic, taking into account chemical, biological and physical exposures, dietary habits, and psychological stress.

- Focus is on separate body parts and their malfunction (as if there were no connection or relation among them).

SPECIALTIES

- Concept of specialization is limited because environmental factors can affect any organ and produce symptoms simultaneously.

- Anatomically demarcated according to the prevailing Cartesian view, i.e., each specialty devoted to one organ only, particularly the division between psychiatry and internal medicine.

THERAPIES

- Avoidance of environmental and dietary offenders, use of nutritional supplements, detoxification, desensitization and neutralization; preventative and cost-effective.

- Primarily pharmaceutical drugs and surgery, which may result in side effects and/or iatrogenic (caused by medical intervention) problems while disease process continues; high risk, high cost.

There are some subtle differences between environmental and allopathic medicine, particularly in relation to history taking, the stage at which disease is diagnosed, focus of medical attention, specialization and therapies, as described by Ashford and Miller.* (See previous page.)

*Ashford, Nicholas and Miller, Claudia, Chemical Exposures—Low Levels and High Stakes, Van Nostrand Reinhold, N.Y., 1991

PRINCIPLES AND PRACTICE OF ENVIRONMENTAL MEDICINE

A specific environmentally oriented medical history (EOMH) is one of the most important factors in the recognition of environmentally triggered diseases. An EOMH relates physical or psychological signs and symptoms to a patient's environmental exposures at home, work or school, different seasons or effects on diet. For example:

- If a patient develops a headache while in the basement, think about an excess of mold from a leaking or flooded basement or fumes from a faulty furnace or stored chemicals.
- Increased symptoms during a specific time of year, influenced by seasons.
- Getting hyper after a school lunch or birthday party.
- Getting tired and sleepy thirty minutes after a meal.
- Experiencing muscle pain, bruising, extreme fatigue or "flu-like symptoms" after exposure to pesticides.
- Irritation of eyes, nose, breathing problems after newly installed carpets, furniture, renovation, etc.

It has to be remembered that any stressor, even a very local trauma, can affect the entire system, e.g., injury to any one body part can lead to fibromyalgia. This occurs through the response of the ground regulating substance (GRS), the basis of which was introduced to us by the Austrian physiologist, A. Pishinger, in Matrix and Matrix Regulation: Basis for a Holistic Theory in Medicine, 1991, Ed. H. Heine.

There are four categories of environmental factors which may trigger ill health (total body load):

CHEMICAL STRESSORS

- Organic substances such as formaldehyde, phenol, benzene, toluene, xylene, plus many chemicals derived from gas, oil and coal. Chlorinated compounds, including organochlorides, pesticides, chloroform, pentachlorophenols, polychlorinated biphenols (PCB) and various herbicides such as 2, 4-D and other pesticides.
- Inorganic substances such as mercury, lead, cadmium, aluminum, asbestos, chlorine, nitrous oxides, sulfur dioxide, ozone, copper, nickel, illegal drugs, tobacco smoke, medications and others.

PHYSICAL STRESSORS

- Heat, cold, weather cycles, noise, positive and negative ions, electromagnetic radiation (full range of the light spectrum), ionizing radiation (radioactivity from x-ray, atomic explosions, reactor accidents, food irradiation, radon gas).

BIOLOGICAL STRESSORS

- Bacteria, viruses, fungi (molds), parasites, foods, animal dander, dust and pollens from trees, grasses and weeds.

PSYCHOLOGICAL STRESSORS

- Any prolonged psychological stress in the family (alcoholism, sexual abuse, family disruption, prolonged sickness of a family member, etc.), or at work (overwork, poor relationships, job loss, etc.); a death in the family, loss due to fire or bankruptcy and other emotional events can trigger unfavourable body responses. These factors are real and can't be overlooked or neglected during therapy.

On the other hand, psychological stress can not only be considered a single cause of prolonged environmental sickness, but can also aggravate or compound existing environmental stress. Additional or secondary psychological stress can also occur when family or medical staff, employers or insurance companies, negate or reject contributing environmental factors. A detailed EOMH will sort out the type of stress involved, as improvement will not occur unless both the stress and the causative environmental factors are dealt with.

PSYCHO-NEURO-ENDOCRINO-IMMUNOLOGY

It is very artificial to divide diseases into psychosomatic and somatic conditions. It has to be remembered that anything that affects the body can also affect the mind, and vice versa. After all, man-made chemicals in minute exposures do affect the central nervous system function as well as other bodily systems. Furthermore, body systems such as the central nervous system, immune endocrine system, etc., communicate with each other through special neuropeptides circulating in the blood. The diagram below represents the interrelationship between the environment and the body.

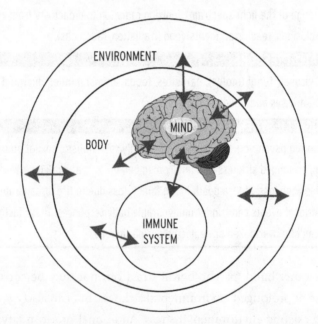

The interactions between immune system, body, mind, and environment.

Source: Cunningham, Alastair J., Mind, Body and Immune Response,
Psychoneuro-immunology, Edited by Robert Ader, Academic Press, Inc., 1981.

TYPES OF EXPOSURES

One of the most important factors in today's chronic degenerative diseases is low-level exposure to chemicals, which causes chemical sensitivity in suffering patients. Chemical sensitivity is defined as an adverse reaction to low, accumulative levels of toxic chemicals, which are usually believed to be at "safe levels." Practically anything we eat, breathe or touch can trigger adverse reactions in a sensitive individual. These reactions can occur as a result of exposure to both natural and man-made chemicals.

The diversity of the manifestations of reactions to chemicals depends upon:

- The pharmacological nature and the toxicity of the substance (more toxic, less toxic, neutral)
- The tissue or organs of the body involved (different symptoms from different organs)
- The age of the patient (newborn, youngest and oldest are most affected)
- The susceptibility of the exposed individual (state of nutrition at the time of exposure, genetic makeup)
- The length of time of exposure and the amount of body stress
- Synergism between different chemicals or their metabolites.

Type of exposure could include:

- Massive (acute): industrial accidents (e.g., Bhopal, India, 1984), wartime exposure (nerve gas, Agent Orange, defoliant herbicides used in the Vietnam War during 1967 to 1968, mix of chemicals, vaccines and depleted uranium—Gulf War, 1991)
- Chronic exposure: takes place when there is chronic accumulation of toxins at work, home, or school (e.g. repeated use of pesticides, painting, cleaning products, renovation supplies)
- Chronic use of antibiotics.

Routes of exposure:

- Lungs, through inhalation of a substance
- Gastrointestinal tract, through ingestion
- Skin, due to touching and absorption, e.g., solvents.

CHANGING FACES OF SENSITIVITY (NO, YOU WON'T "OUTGROW" IT)

Environmental sensitivities and allergies have many faces. Manifestations, signs and symptoms during the life of the affected individual change and intertwine. Parents of a child suffering from allergies and sensitivities are often told that the child will "outgrow" the problem. As a matter of fact, the child never does. I was once memorably told by my professor of pediatrics that we "outgrow our pants, but not the disease."

The following are common symptoms in a sensitive individual throughout the course of his/her life from infancy through adolescence to adulthood:

CHILDREN

IN UTERO

- the baby is excessively active in utero, has hiccups and/or is very, very quiet
- the expectant mother, meanwhile, has cravings for specific foods which she indulges, and which in turn sensitize the baby in utero, e.g., milk, sugar

INFANT

- colicky baby, frequent changes of formula
- constant stuffiness and/or runny nose
- eczema
- rocking and banging the head against the crib
- difficulties in falling asleep and waking up
- chronic and recurrent ear infections
- excessive perspiration, drooling

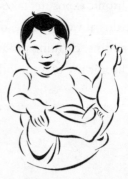

TODDLER

- leg cramps or "growing pains"
- not able to cuddle, constant wiggling
- temper tantrums, biting
- removing clothes
- sleep problems
- vomiting clear white mucous
- sleeping a lot—child's narcolepsy
- chronic respiratory infections and recurrent use of antibiotics

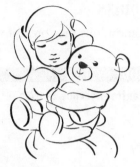

PRESCHOOL AND SCHOOL AGE

- runny nose and stuffiness
- breathing problems, asthma, bronchitis
- constant diarrhea or constipation, bedwetting, rushing to the bathroom
- excessive gas, belly aches, bad breath
- tired or excessively active, learning problems

ADOLESCENT

- chronic tiredness, emotional instability, irritability
- depression, suicidal tendencies
- muscle aches, headache
- bowel problems
- forgetfulness, inability to concentrate
- alcoholism
- obesity, anorexia nervosa

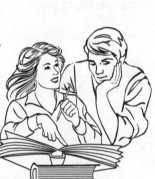

PRINCIPLES

ADULTS

Some adults may present with any number of the following symptoms:

BODY SYSTEM	SYMPTOM	
Central Nervous System	fatigue	headache
	tension	memory loss
	confusion	depression
	hallucinations	dizziness
	hyperactivity	numbness
	sleep disorders	tremors
Gastrointestinal System	heartburn	bloating
	nausea	constipation/diarrhea
Hematological System	high or low platelets	bruising
	anemia	leucopenia
Genitourinary System	frequency	infertility
	inability to void	infection of urinary tract
	urgency to urinate	interstitial cystitis
	prostate problems	
Musculoskeletal System	joint pain	muscle pain
	backaches	muscle spasms
	swollen limbs	muscle twitching
	muscle weakness	
Respiratory System	frequent colds	asthma
	bronchitis	heavy chest
	shortness of breath	sighing respiration
ENT System	nasal stuffiness	earaches
	sinus infections	ear infections
	watery eyes	
Skin	flushing	rashes
	eczema	hives
	cold extremities	
Cardiovascular System	rapid heart beat	irregular heart beat
	skip beats	hypertension/hypotension

PRINCIPLES OF ENVIRONMENTAL MEDICINE

To understand environmental aspects of health and disease we must look at the four principles involved in the process: total load, masking phenomenon, bipolarity, and biological individuality.

Total load (total body burden)

Total load consists of past and present physical, chemical, biological contaminants in food, air and water, as well as the emotional state of the individual. You can compare total body burden to a container—you can only fill it to capacity. Anything above capacity causes spillover or, in other words, allergic symptoms and ultimately sickness. Another image to keep in mind is the straw that breaks the camel's back.

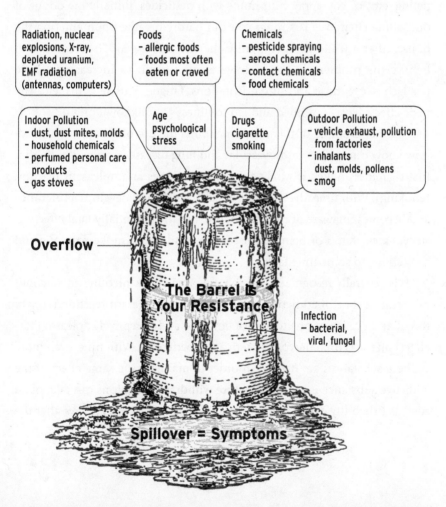

Radiation, nuclear explosions, X-ray, depleted uranium, EMF radiation (antennas, computers)

Foods
- allergic foods
- foods most often eaten or craved

Chemicals
- pesticide spraying
- aerosol chemicals
- contact chemicals
- food chemicals

Indoor Pollution
- dust, dust mites, molds
- household chemicals
- perfumed personal care products
- gas stoves

Age psychological stress

Drugs cigarette smoking

Outdoor Pollution
- vehicle exhaust, pollution from factories
- inhalants
  dust, molds, pollens
- smog

Overflow

The Barrel is Your Resistance

Infection
- bacterial, viral, fungal

Spillover = Symptoms

Masking Phenomenon (adaptation, tolerance, addiction)

The human body is brilliantly designed with a complex and comprehensive network of psychoneuro-endocrino-immunological mechanisms for maintaining good health and equilibrium, which is homeostasis. Stressors are handled through the process of adaptation, which allows for compensatory physiological responses (e.g., detoxification) to the chronic stress of environmental challenges. Illness occurs when the adaptive process becomes exhausted.

Adaptation, through *"masking,"* makes it difficult sometimes to see the connection between a particular exposure and symptoms. For example, you renovate or move into a new home—fresh paint, refinished floors, new carpeting, etc., or you spray your home with pesticides. Initially the odour of outgassing chemicals is strong; you can hardly breathe upon entering the house. After a while you get used to the smell or use air "fresheners" and believe the problem is gone. However, you begin to increasingly have headaches, eye, nose and throat irritations, fatigue, muscle pains, etc. The toxic effects have continued and led to illness "of unknown origin."

Another example of this phenomenon is the use of tobacco, which we now know can lead to cardiovascular and lung disease, among others. That first cigarette smoked is rarely enjoyed and causes an unpleasant reaction (choking). With time, the smoker (or family member) develops a **tolerance** and becomes unaware of even the odour, but the potentially fatal effects of smoking cigarettes or being exposed to second-hand smoke continue and only show up some time later.

It is generally recognized that the use of narcotics, nicotine and alcohol can create a state of **addiction**. After an initial unpleasant reaction (cough, throat and eye irritation) tolerance develops and deceptively "pleasurable" effects on the central nervous system are experienced. With time, even more of these substances are needed in order to maintain the same effect. If the addictive substance is removed, severe withdrawal reactions can take place such as irritability, fatigue, moodiness, headache, etc. Several days after the withdrawal reaction, the individual remains hypersensitive to secondary smoke or the smell of alcohol, with a recurrence of the initial unpleasant reactions upon exposure but still a strong need to continue the habit. **At this point, the individual can tough it out, kick the habit and regain health** or he/she can return to the habit, and "feel good" or "relieved," while damage to the heart, brain, lungs, liver and other organs continues from the toxic effects.

The same masking phenomenon can occur with low-level exposure to chemical toxins. This has been documented in studies on factory employees exposed to solvents, nitroglycerin, welding fumes, cotton, grain and other organic dusts. Workers unknowingly experienced withdrawal symptoms on the weekend and often preferred to return to work, where these symptoms cleared upon re-exposure to the substances. However, years of exposure led to demonstrable pathological changes in the central nervous, endocrine, cardiovascular and immune systems, resulting in disease. Low-level exposures over a long period of time can be as harmful as acute exposure, and only the time factor makes a difference. **Early intervention (avoidance, making the workplace safe, detoxification treatment) can prevent the development of chronic illness.**

Something similar can happen with foods consumed every day (breads, sweets, coffee, milk, etc.). The individual learns to eat a particular food repeatedly at whatever interval of time is required to feel satisfied. When the meal or snack of this food is postponed or missed, withdrawal symptoms such as fatigue, depression, irritability, headache, etc. occur. Consciously or not, a "fix" is needed. By eating the masking food regularly, a gratification effect is maintained. A typical pattern may include cereal with milk for breakfast, coffee and danish/muffin for a mid-morning break, cheese sandwich with milk or pop for lunch, afternoon coffee and snack bar break, pasta for dinner with a sweet dessert, milk and cookie at bedtime. Patients often can't understand that commonly eaten and well-liked foods can be the cause of their ill health, since food is considered beneficial, not harmful.

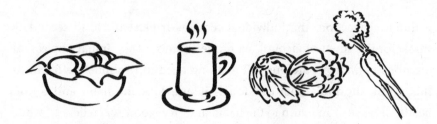

It is not known how we become addicted to foods (see page 141). However, foods consist not only of protein, fats and carbohydrates, but also of natural chemicals (phenolic food compounds and even morphine). Daily indulgent consumption of a limited number of foods can cause not only nutritional deficiency, but also sensitization and allergy. This creates immune complexes that can cause inflammation of target organs in susceptible individuals, leading to various symptoms. For example, wheat products can be a factor in irritable bowel syndrome for one person, migraines in another, arthritis in a third, eczema in a fourth, etc. Foods can also cause psychological symptoms in the genetically susceptible individual.

Physicians, poorly trained in understanding adaptation mechanisms, or not trained at all, do not connect cause with effect. For example, a patient comes in complaining of irritable bowel syndrome, arthritic pains or migraine, etc. If the doctor doesn't know that foods can cause these symptoms, the complaints will only receive a label and medication offering symptomatic relief, while the disease process continues uninterrupted. In another instance,

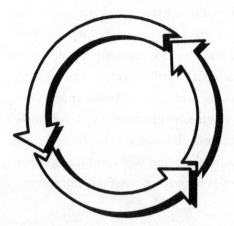

a patient for some reason has been unable to have that favourite food for a couple of days (due to an illness, an operation, a trip, a diet). Withdrawal reactions set in and the individual feels sick but doesn't know why. The patient then goes to the doctor, who wouldn't make the connection to the food because she doesn't know what questions to ask and because the food wasn't ingested recently. In the case of a diet, the individual may happily return to eating that favourite food convinced that eating it makes him feel better. The addiction continues and, as any addiction, can carry with it ill consequences.

A simple way to **unmask** sensitivities is to avoid an offending substance in any form and related food family members (e.g., all grains, all dairy) for five to seven days. Withdrawal reactions will take place within the first two or three days, after which there is total freedom from any symptoms relating to the offending substance. Upon re-exposure to the suspect substance, the body will give clear-cut, reproducible reactions. The disappearance of symptoms during a longer period of time, when there is no contact with an offending substance, and a rapid recurrence after re-exposure to the same substance is the basis for **challenge** or **provocative** tests, which prove cause and effect.

When exposures to toxic or allergic substances continue and are compounded by the other environmental factors listed earlier, the adaptive mechanisms become exhausted. While your body is brilliantly designed to, under the right circumstances, detoxify and/or fight disease, overload can cause damage to the detox and immune systems and the disease process can then fully develop. **The encouraging news is that, with education and foresight, you can practice preventative medicine.** This does, however, require some self-discipline and a sense of responsibility; moreover the benefits are not only improved health, but also regaining control over it. This in turn leads to higher self-esteem and subsequent physical and psychological well-being. It's all connected. Taking it a step further and introducing this concept to the whole family may also benefit other members. Children's health could improve, along with their listening and learning skills.

BIPOLARITY (BIPHASIC PATTERN OF REACTION)
Dr. Theron Randolph,* the father of Clinical Ecology, observing thousands of patients in environmental units reacting to different substances (foods,

PRINCIPLES

inhalants, chemicals), noted that at the beginning of a reaction, the patient showed stimulatory symptoms which could last varying lengths of time (period of development of adaptation to the substance). After the stimulatory phase, the patient showed signs of depression (withdrawal reaction as a loss of adaptation or maladaptation response). The graph below shows that phenomenon.

Randolph, Theron. Environmental Medicine—Beginnings and Biographies of Clinical Ecology. *Citizen Printing, Fort Collins, Colorado, 1987.*

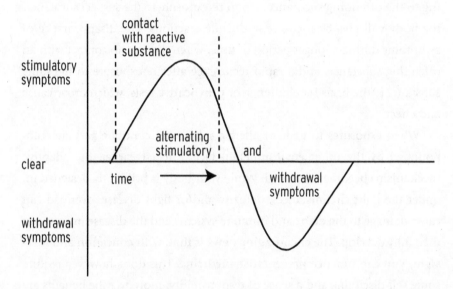

(From O'Banion, D.R., Ecological and Nutritional Treatment of Health Disorders, 1981, p. 68. Charles C. Thomas, Publisher, Springfield, Illinois)

Often the frequency of the stimulatory and depressive phase depends on the amount of contact with the substance. The amplitude of these reactions depends on the characteristics of the substance and the individual reactivity of the patient.

Many levels of these reactions are characteristic of CNS manifestations such as excitability, nervousness, confusion and depression. Levels +1 and +2 are reactions characteristic of the adaptive response and the patient usually does not seek help from a doctor. The beginning of depressive (withdrawal) reactions at levels −1 and −2 gives systemic symptoms such as tiredness, difficulties in concentrating, headache, etc. and/or local reactions, including bronchitis, asthma or diarrhea, which prompt the patient to see a doctor. Therefore, after stimulatory phase +2, the depressive phase may develop at levels −2 or −3, which is the withdrawal reaction. It is interesting to note that the tendency toward psychiatric types of reaction manifest at levels +4 and −4 and are at the peaks of the sinusoid curve, while classical allergy manifestations are at levels −1 and −2 (See Table on page 48.).

ENVIRONMENTAL CONTROL UNITS

The concept of Environmental Control Units (ECU) was first developed by Dr. Theron Randloph and brought to a state of the art level by Dr. William Rea of Dallas, Texas. It is a segregated inpatient ward, constructed especially with no outgassing materials (ceramics, steel, porcelain on steel), special ventilation, air filtration and positive air pressure to ensure 100% control over the indoor air quality. An ECU is the ideal place for a patient to be properly diagnosed, the appropriate cause of symptoms to be established and appropriate therapy instituted. The graph on page 49 depicts symptoms of an individual before and after entering an Environmental Control Unit (ECU).

Very subtle reactions can be difficult to observe in a patient's home or regular hospital because there are many factors contributing to the reactions (natural gas, perfumes, tobacco smoke, paints, solvents, foods, coffee, allergens such as molds, trees, etc.), which can affect the patient simultaneously (time period A). Differentiation of cause and effect can be difficult to determine.

In order to exclude interfering environmental factors or "background noise," it is important to place a patient in an ECU, where the number of parameters influencing a patient is minimal. In time period B, a patient enters the unit and starts to fast, consuming only well tolerated spring

Environmental-personal interrelationships

	INTERMITTENT RESPONSES	LEVELS	SUSTAINED RESPONSES
Specifically adapted stimulatory levels	MANIA (agitation, excitement, blackouts, with or without convulsions)	++++	DRUG ADDICTION (both natural and synthetic)
	HYPOMANIA (hyperresponsiveness, anxiety, panic reactions, mental lapses)	+++	ALCOHOLISM (addictive drinking)
	HYPERACTIVITY (restless legs, insomnia, aggressive, forceful behaviour)	++	OBESITY (addictive eating)
	STIMULATION (active, self-centered with suppressed symptoms)	+	ABSENT COMPLAINTS (the desired way to feel)
	BEHAVIOUR ON AN EVEN KEEL, AS IN HOMEOSTASIS	0	**BEHAVIOUR ON AN EVEN KEEL**
Specifically maladapted withdrawal levels	LOCALIZED PHYSICAL ECOLOGIC MANIFESTATIONS (rhinitis, bronchitis, asthma, dermatitis, gastrointestinal, genitourinary syndromes)	–	IMPAIRED SENSES OF TASTE AND SMELL, MENIERE'S SYNDROME
	SYSTEMIC PHYSICAL ECOLOGIC MANIFESTATIONS (fatigue, headache, myalgia, arthralgia, arthritis, edema, tachycardia, arrhythmia)	– –	SMALL VESSEL VASCULITIS, HYPERTENSION, COLLAGEN DISEASES
	BRAIN EFFECTS—MODERATELY ADVANCED CEREBRAL SYNDROMES (mood changes, irritability, impaired thinking, reading ability & memory)	– – –	MENTAL CONFUSION AND OBFUSCATION, MOROSE INEBRIATION
	DEPRESSION—ADVANCED CEREBRAL & BEHAVIOURAL SYNDROMES (confabulation, hallucinosis, obsessions, delusions & temporary amnesia)	– – – –	DEMENTIA, STUPOR, COMA, CATATONIA, RESIDUAL AMNESIA

Randolph T, Moss R. An Alternative Approach To Allergies. J. B.Lippincot Co., 1980

water. There is cessation of previous exposures, withdrawal effects (headache, nausea, etc.), and symptoms continue for some time usually four to seven days, until patients feel 100% normal, the baseline.

In time period C, single challenges to suspect incitants are administered. The effect of each substance can be assessed and measured individually and a *cause* and *effect* relationship can be established.

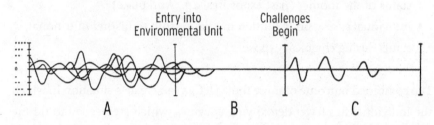

Ashford Nicholas A, Miller Claudia S, Chemical Exposures, Low Levels and High Stakes, 2nd edition. Van Nostrand Reinhold, 1998.

In an Environmental Control Unit, specialized tests can be performed in specially constructed booths, where the concentration of any chemical can be precisely measured and the effect of that chemical on the patient can be objectively assessed by carefully monitoring signs and symptoms.

It is mandatory that any physician practicing Environmental Medicine provides a very clean, scent-free office, especially the testing area, to assure accurate test results.

The effects of chemicals, foods or inhalants on a patient's health should be examined and considered before excluding in favour of a diagnosis of a mental or psychological disorder, as is often the case.

BIOCHEMICAL INDIVIDUALITY

This final principle is key to the understanding of environmental medicine. No two individuals are exactly alike; biological individuality is the basis for our individual susceptibility. We have individual needs of amounts of vitamins, minerals, enzymes, protein, fat, and carbohydrates for appropriate function of our organs and particularly our CNS and immune system, so that we are able to respond to environmental factors that we are challenged with on a daily basis. There are three conditions upon which our biological individuality depends:

- Genetic makeup of the fetus (result of the parents' genes)
- Health of the mother, toxic burden during pregnancy, nutritional status of the mother (past exposures, e.g., workplace)
- Individual's toxic body burden in relationship to his/her nutritional status during chemical exposure.

The combined outcome of these three factors can create a situation in which the individual has fewer detoxifying enzymes, which are needed to rid the body of toxins. If the body is unable to detoxify fast enough, a situation is set up which can allow a serious disease to develop. There are over 2000 so-called inborn errors of metabolism (genetic metabolic defects), and the number is growing. They are a "time bomb" only awaiting the opportune moment when environmental triggers elicit their expression.

In summary, the development of an environmental sensitivity looks something like this:

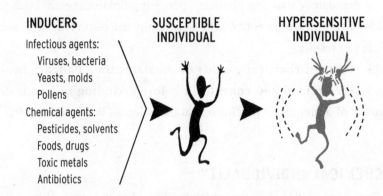

INDUCERS	SUSCEPTIBLE INDIVIDUAL	HYPERSENSITIVE INDIVIDUAL

Infectious agents:
  Viruses, bacteria
  Yeasts, molds
  Pollens
Chemical agents:
  Pesticides, solvents
  Foods, drugs
  Toxic metals
  Antibiotics

According to recent research of Ashford and Miller, there have emerged four major groups of people suffering from chemical sensitivities:

GROUP	NATURE OF EXPOSURE	DEMOGRAPHICS
Industrial Workers	Acute and chronic exposure to industrial chemicals	Primarily males; blue collar; 20 to 65 years old
Tight-Building Occupants	Off-gassing from construction materials, office equipment or supplies; tobacco smoke; inadequate ventilation	Females more than males; white-collar office workers and professionals; 20 to 65 years old; schoolchildren
Contaminated Communities	Toxic waste sites, aerial pesticide spraying, ground water contamination, air contamination by nearby industry and other community exposures	All ages, male and female; children or infants may be affected first or most; pregnant women with possible effects on fetuses; middle to lower class
Individuals	Heterogeneous; indoor air (domestic), consumer products, drugs, and pesticides	70–80% females; 50% 30 to 50 years old (Johnson and Rea, 1989); white, middle to upper middle class and professionals

Ashford, Nicholas and Miller, Claudia, Chemical Exposures—Low Levels and High Stakes, *Van Nostrand Reinhold, N.Y., 1991)*

Multiple Chemical Sensitivity (MCS)

The following are consensus criteria for the diagnosis of MCS, which were formulated by researchers and clinicians with experience in the study, evaluation, diagnosis and/or care of adults and children with chemical sensitivity disorders:

1. *"The symptoms are reproducible with (repeated chemical) exposure."*
2. *"The condition is chronic."*
3. *"Low levels of exposure (lower than previously or commonly tolerated) result in manifestations of the syndrome."*

4. *"The symptoms improve or resolve when the incitants are removed."*
5. *"Responses occur to multiple chemically unrelated substances."*
6. *(Added in 1999): Symptoms involve multiple organ systems.*

The only other explicit consensus to have been published on MCS was a 1994 statement of the American Lung Association, the American Medical Association, the US Environmental Protection Agency, and the US Consumer Product Safety Commission, to state that "complaints (of MCS) should not be dismissed as psychogenic, and a thorough workup is essential." It is recommended that MCS be diagnosed whenever all six of the consensus criteria are met, along with any other disorders that may also be present, such as asthma, allergy, migraine, chronic fatigue syndrome (CFS), and fibromyalgia (FM).

Multiple Chemical Sensitivity: A 1999 Consensus, Archives of Environmental Medicine; May/June 1999 (Vol. 54 (No.3))

Remember the case history of each person is very individual. While the causes of reactions and symptoms will differ, it is the total body load that must be brought under control, and awareness and knowledge is the first step towards making a positive change.

The aim of this handbook is to provide you with information about the elements that can affect an individual's health, and to offer management techniques.

MEDICAL OFFICE

The ideal medical office will try to achieve the best air quality using chemical and particulate filtration systems with appropriate air exchange, humidity levels and positive air pressure. The floors will be ceramic or hardwood with a non-toxic finish. If cost precludes ceramic or porcelain steel walls, plaster walls are preferable to drywall and painted with low outgassing paint.

Full-spectrum incandescent lighting is preferable to fluorescent, certainly in the testing areas, as fluorescent lighting can cause reactions, particularly seizures, in some patients. Furniture should be metal or already outgassed wood. Administrative areas should be separate from testing, and lab areas should be vented. All supplies should be stored away from patient exposure. Staff should not be using any scented products.

These arrangements make everyone happier and healthier and able to work and concentrate better. Patients generally feel better right away, relaxed and confident. Any testing to be carried out is easier and more precise in a clean environment. Patients are provided with a model of the value of investing in proper air ventilation and filtration.

A patient who is suffering from outdoor allergy or chemical exposure symptoms should be able to feel relief from such symptoms just by sitting in such an office for half an hour.

The Initial Investigation Period:

- Consultation with the doctor, including detailed past, present, and environmental medical history, system review, past surgeries, adverse reactions to medication and/or supplements, occupational and/or school history, dietary analysis, including patterns of eating, and physical examination;
- Blood and urine analysis, sputum, mouth, throat, and vaginal swabs, pulmonary function tests, etc. as deemed necessary by the doctor for the individual patient;
- Testing for food, inhalant, and/or chemical sensitivities;
- Counseling (individual or group with trained staff member) involving office orientation, four-day rotation diet, addressing water and environmental control techniques;
- Follow-up visit with the doctor.

Laboratory Testing:

Most laboratories, and particularly those in Canada, are not able to offer precise tests measuring biochemical, nutritional and immunological status of the patient. Most laboratories use outdated methods and tests, which are not able to detect and measure subtle biochemical changes. This unfortunate situation leads doctors, insurance companies and the Workers' Compensation Board to label the patient, in whom nothing "abnormal" is found but who nevertheless reports multi-systemic complaints, as suffering from "psychosomatic" illness. This is an unfair label for many genuinely sick individuals, particularly since there is no test to prove psychosomatic disease, but this diagnosis often seems to be easier than finding the cause of illness in our sociopolitical environment.

There are laboratories available in the United States that perform more sophisticated tests, but they are often dismissed by some critics whose vested interests lie elsewhere as being "entrepreneurial" and "non-scientific." Despite the critics, there are some very reliable laboratories that can assess the nutritional status of the patient. These laboratories are licensed at both the federal and state levels, and the test results are accepted by the United States medical insurance companies.

Some of the specialized tests performed include:
- Measurement of intracellular minerals and levels of vitamins, amino acids and lipids
- Assessment of oxidative damage to the cell
- Assessment of detoxifying ability
- Measurement of toxic levels of chemicals in blood or fat tissue such as solvents, chlorinated pesticides, herbicides, PCBs, etc.
- Assessment of immune status, measurement of immune functions, specific antibodies (formaldehyde, plastics), auto antibodies (CNS, peripheral nervous system), etc.
- Neuropsychological testing.

After the initial period, you may require:

- Additional visits with the doctor
- Retesting of the allergy treatment extract—seasonally, for injectable (6 weeks prior to the beginning of an antigen season); upon completion of your first bottle of sublingual, and then whenever necessary; if you have recently experienced a viral infection, it may sometimes alter your body's response and you may require a different extract; or if you suspect your treatment is not working (symptoms have returned).
- Additional counseling (at your request)
- Detoxification, I.V. therapy, immune stimulation
- Referral to other physicians.

Environmental Office Policies

While each individual office will set its own policies, generally speaking, out of care and concern for patients and staff, individuals with tobacco or perfume odours or otherwise scented clothing will be asked to leave the office. Some physicians do not accept patients who smoke or whose family members smoke, and require that the patient and family members are smoke-free for three months. Tobacco smoke and secondary smoke cause and compound many health problems.

Policies regarding testing and procedures, serum ordering and re-ordering, other services, payment, etc., will be at the discretion of the individual office.

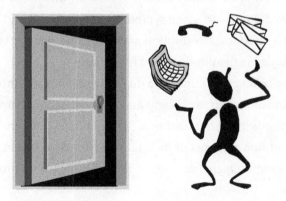

TYPES OF TESTING

Various forms of testing for allergies or sensitivities are used based on individual needs. Most commonly used are Serial Dilution Endpoint Titration (SDEPT) and Provocation/Neutralization. These tests were pioneered by Drs. Carleton Lee, Herbert Rinkel and Joseph Miller. It was found that introducing various dilutions of antigens intradermally not only produced a whealing response on the skin, but also general signs and symptoms. Sublingual testing was pioneered by Dr. Lawrence Dickey. All these methods can be used to test for food, inhalant and chemical allergies or sensitivities.

1. **Provocative/Neutralization (P/N):** The patient is systematically exposed to a series of dilutions of a suspect antigen extract. When symptoms appear (are provoked), a neutralizing dose is found and used in treatment. Dilutions of an antigen can be administered:

   a) **Intradermally**—into the skin.

   Using a syringe, a precise amount of measured antigen is injected into the skin producing a 4mm wheal. During the ten minutes after the injection, signs and symptoms are recorded. After ten minutes, the pulse is recorded and the size of the wheal is measured. The first strongest negative wheal, with no symptom, is often the neutralizing dilution and is used for treatment (Miller technique).

   b) **Sublingually**—under the tongue.

   Using a dropper or syringe, a precise quantity of measured antigen extract is dropped under the tongue, held for thirty seconds, then swallowed. Pulse, signs and symptoms are measured and recorded every five minutes. The dilution after which no signs or symptoms are recorded is the dilution used for therapy.

   Provocative testing often uncovers the cause of chronic symptoms in a very convincing way to the patient and is an educational experience for patients observing the reactions. Some patients can hardly believe that even minute amounts of their favourite foods or fragrances can create the symptoms that are part of their chronic health problems.

2. **Serial Dilution End-Point Titration (SDEPT):** Using a syringe, a precise quantity of the suspect antigen is injected into the skin, producing a 4mm wheal. After ten minutes, the growth of the wheal is measured. Testing continues until two positive wheals are produced. A delayed reaction may occur; therefore, all patients treated in this manner must inform the office the next day to have their arm checked by a technician. Since wheal growth is the only determining factor for this technique, several antigens can be tested at the same time.

   SDEPT testing is time-consuming but precise, and discovers the safe and exact dose that is used for desensitization treatment. It is fundamentally different from the standard allergy prick testing and serum preparation used by most so-called traditional allergists. It is not only precise and reliable, but also very safe with no reports of any fatalities.

3. **Prick Test:** This test is primarily used by conventional allergists and is only useful as a basic test for inhalant allergy. A drop of undiluted antigen is placed on the patient's forearm or back. A prick of the skin through the drop is performed using a needle. Skin response is read thirty minutes after the prick.

   The prick test is really only a guide to existing sensitivities, but is not able to define a safe point at which to start immunotherapy. This is the reason for which sometimes-fatal reactions can develop during immunotherapy based on use of the prick test.

   For all three tests, P/N, SDEPT and Prick, a negative control with normal saline and a positive control with histamine are performed at the same time.

4. **Radio-Allergo-Sorbent (RAST) Test:** This is a blood test and has good diagnostic values, specifically for IgE-mediated allergies (primarily inhalants).

5. **Electrodermal Testing (EDT):** This testing technique is based upon bioenergetic regulatory theory. Various electrodermal equipment can be used, including Dermatron according to Voll, Listen, Best, Entero,

Vega, Biomeridian MSA-21, etc. Newer models are computerized. Practitioners use them to assess stress conditions of tissues or organs to a variety of substances and assess patients for sensitivities, intolerances, etc. All measure galvanic skin response by employing a minute electrical current conducted through a probe to responsive acupuncture points. Every substance assessed has a unique vibrational characteristic or electromagnetic wave, which is conducted by a weak electrical signal through the device, affecting the autonomic nervous system of the individual to increase or decrease sweat production. These changes cause an increase or decrease in skin resistance, which is recorded by the galvanometer. In the case of environmental medicine screening, neutralizing doses can be quickly and easily determined and then confirmed sublingually. The method is time-efficient, accurate, and exposes the patient to less stress than, for example, invasive needle testing. It is particularly useful for highly sensitive patients and for children.

None of these tests provide a medical diagnosis. They are used for screening and for gathering information.

www.healthy.net/aaabem/EAV/earexplained.htm

TREATMENTS

There is no easy solution to improvement of the patient's allergies and/or sensitivities; nevertheless, better management is the key to enhancement of health. The principles of Environmental Medicine can be applied to the treatment of many chronic, degenerative diseases with resultant improvement of overall well-being. It empowers the patient and provides the necessary tools to improve and maintain optimal health.

In the practice of Environmental Medicine, in the absence of any acute problems, which require immediate intervention, the emphasis is placed on **education, diet, nutrition, detoxification, oral or I.V. chelation for heavy metals or cardiovascular and degenerative diseases, exercise/relaxation** and **immunotherapy**. Prevention is preferable to prescribing countless symptom-suppressing and side-effect-causing pharmaceutical drugs. However, some pharmaceutical drugs are used in acute cases or chronic situations until appropriate recovery can take place with an effective nutritional and detoxification prescription. In the case of Stealth Infections (see page 292), longer-term use of antibiotics with appropriate probiotic supplementation is a necessity.

What the patient must realize is that there is **no magic pill**. Maintaining good health and prevention of disease entails effort and self-discipline. The patient must take responsibility for his/her own health and that of their family. Family support in patient efforts is also crucial.

The following is a short description of treatment areas. More details are provided in the Management Section beginning on page 181 of this guide.

Education
- how environmental factors can affect the individual
- sources of inhalants and chemicals at home, work and/or school
- environmental control at home (creating a safe and healthy home)
- food as a cause of symptoms or adverse reactions
- organic versus inorganic food
- safe water supply
- detoxification
- understanding allergy, anaphylaxis and sensitivities

Diet and Nutrition
- Four-Day Rotation Diet
- emphasis on organic foods
- correction of nutritional deficiencies
- enhancement of detoxification and immune system
- use of tolerable vitamin and mineral supplements, oral and I.V.
- elimination of "junk food"
- use of safe water for drinking and cooking

Exercise/Relaxation
- regular and moderate exercise at least three times per week
- adequate oxygenation through proper breathing
- positive thinking, meditation
- psychological support if necessary

IMMUNOTHERAPY

Antigen Therapy
Allergy treatment extracts are an injectable or sublingual dilution of the antigen which testing has shown to be the most effective for control of symptoms for the individual. For each antigen that aggravates an individual, there is a dilution of the same antigen that will improve tolerance and neutralize symptoms.

What Are They For?
To improve an individual's tolerance to items that are difficult to avoid, and to desensitize the individual.

What Else Do They Contain?
Antigens can be diluted in water, glycerin, or a phenolated saline solution. Phenol-free antigens are also available to accommodate the needs of patients who are sensitive to this substance.

Types of Antigen Therapy
I. Injectable: foods, chemicals and inhalants
    a) based on SDEPT, P/N methods
    b) Enzyme Potentiated Desensitization (EPD) (see page 267)—
       a highly diluted mixture of antigens (foods, inhalants and chemicals) mixed with beta glucuronidase enzyme to enhance the desensitization process

II. **Sublingual:** foods, chemicals and inhalants
   a) For individual or mixed substances
   b) for phenolic food compounds (naturally occurring chemicals in the plant kingdom)

How Do I Take Them?

Specific written instructions will be given to the patient when their treatment extract is provided. Generally, if the patient has been tested with needles, then their extract will be injected subcutaneously (under the skin), whereas antigens tested with drops, or on the EDT device, will be taken sublingually (under the tongue).

Antigen injections are usually given once a week in the patient's family doctor's office. If you notice immediate or delayed reactions, **notify** the staff before your next injection and **insist** on a readjustment of the dose based on the written instructions given. If reactions persist, arrange for retesting.

If you require injections more often than once per week or you are unable to make weekly trips for injections, you can give them to yourself after receiving **full instructions in your doctor's office**. The injections based on these precise and individually tested dilutions (SDEPT / P/N) are perfectly safe to self-administer, unlike regular allergy shots, for which dilutions are arbitrarily and blindly defined.

With EPD, injections are given once every two months during the first year, once every three months in the second year, and then, two or three times a year on an individual basis as a maintenance dose. There is a protocol to follow before the needle is given, during the four critical days around the needle, and after the needle, that involves gastrointestinal preparation, diet, nutritional supplements and environmental control.

PRINCIPLES

How Long Will I Need to Take Them?

Once again, each patient is individual. A great deal depends on the ability to maintain environmental controls and dietary changes. Some patients only need a period of time to become desensitized, others feel better using allergy treatment extracts on a regular but progressively infrequent basis, and still others require daily or weekly treatment to control symptoms. This question is best discussed with your doctor.

What Effect Could Immunnotherapy Have?

- Immediate beneficial effect—neutralization, clearing of symptoms;
- Delayed beneficial effect—within three to six weeks, the patient will be able to tolerate environmental exposures and foods much better;
- Immediate or delayed negative response—more symptoms. If this occurs, discontinue treatment and schedule a retesting appointment.

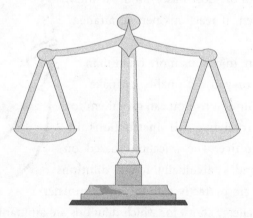

The goal of treatment is to establish balance, or homeostasis.

AUTOGENOUS VACCINES

In some rare cases of patients with chronic urinary tract infections, bronchiec-tasis, chronic bone infections, etc., which do not respond to antibiotics or have developed antibiotic resistance, autogenous vaccine is useful and sometimes even life-saving. It has been mostly used and researched in Europe. Before antibiotics were widely available, this was a major method in Europe to control infections.

A sample from the affected organ is taken (urine, pus, sputum, biopsy, etc.) to test for culture and sensitivity in a lab. If positive, a sample is placed in normal saline, all bacteria killed by heat or radiation, and the solution filtered through a 0.22μ bacterial filter and serially diluted by a factor of 5. Testing using the SDEPT method is carried out. 0.05 cc of the first strongest negative wheal is injected on a daily basis, with an increasing volume of up to 0.5–0.8 cc. Once the first skin reaction is achieved, return to the previous volume with a negative skin response. Continue injecting this volume two times per week for a period of from six weeks to three months. In the major-ity of cases, a complete resolution and healing occurs.

See Resources Section.

Inhalants, Fungi and Molds

Inhalants are airborne particles that we breathe on a daily basis. In fact, it has been stated that every day we breathe two tablespoons of assorted particles. The average individual can deal with these intruders; however, they do add stress to the body. For the allergic person, these inhalants can be a catastrophe as their body copes poorly with them.

For discussion purposes, inhalants can be divided into two groups: indoor and outdoor. Listed below are the common inhalants tested in many environmental medicine or allergy offices.

INDOOR INHALANTS

House Dust (HD)

- A mixture of whatever is floating in the air, including; lint, mites, danders, insect parts, bacteria, food particles, bits of plants and other particulate matter, bacteria, cosmetics, dirt, feathers, wool fibres, molds, and human epidermis;
- The disintegration of household articles also contributes to dust (foam, mattresses, fibres).

Household Insects (HHI)

- Insect parts (scales, wings, bit of hard outer shell);
- Dried secretions from:
  – ant, black fly, cockroach, mosquito, fly.

Animal Dander

- Cats and dogs are the usual offenders, but horses and other animals can also be offenders;
- Dander is particles of hair and skin that cling to the animal's fur;
- A sensitivity can develop at any time;
- Animal saliva and urine can also be a problem;
- Mohair, alpaca, horse hair, feathers and down used for textiles and stuffing may also cause problems.

Dust Mites

- A microscopic relative of ticks and spiders
- Thrive in warm, humid places and feed on human skin scales
- Harmful allergens are found in the house dust mite's fecal pellets
- Lives primarily in bed mattresses, pillows and carpet

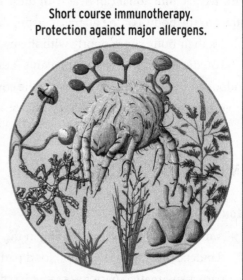

Short course immunotherapy.
Protection against major allergens.

· Tree Pollens · Grass Pollens · Ragweed Pollens
· Mould Spores · House Dust Mite

"Dust Mite." Picture courtesy of Bencard Allergy Laboratories.

MOLDS AND FUNGI

Facts

- The inhalation of spores (reproductive part of fungi) causes a reaction in sensitive individuals. Once inhaled, spores can enter the digestive and circulatory system, and therefore symptoms can be wide-ranging.
- Fungi fall into 2 categories:
  yeast: single-celled, divide to form clusters.
  mold: multi-celled, grow as branching threads that form colonies.
- These simple organisms take their food from plants, animals, decayed matter, paint, paste and human skin.
- Fungi can grow almost anywhere, indoors and out. They particularly like dark, damp places, and can survive at low temperatures. Some can even live through the first frost of the winter. **The only time outdoor levels are low is when there has been snow on the ground for five or more days.**

Molds tested in an environmental medicine office are those most commonly found in the given geographical area. Any mold species or combination can be tested and treated. They can include:

- **Alternaria Tenuis:** found on plants and plant material. It has been stated to be one of the most common causes of symptoms due to allergy to airborne mold spores.
- **Aspergillus Fumigatus:** found in soil, damp hay, grains, sausage, fruit.
- **Hormodendrum (Cladosporium):** found in decomposing plants, leather, rubber, cloth, paper and other wood products. It is abundant in air samples and released after rains, and when the weather is damp.
- **Penicillium Notatum:** found in soil, fruits, breads, cheese and other foods. A mutant strain of this is used for the medication, penicillin.

Note: Occasionally it is necessary to grow a mold from your own home environment in order to diagnose and treat your specific symptoms.

INHALANTS

- T.O.E.: A combination of three pathogenic fungi:
  - Tricophyton
  - Oidomycetis (Candida)
  - Epidermophyton
- Candida: lives on mucous membranes within the human body and on the skin.

Sources of Airborne Molds in Homes

- Damp rooms with poor ventilation, e.g. flooded, leaky basements, kitchens, shower areas of bathrooms
- Carpeting
- Closets, drawers, hampers with damp or unwashed clothing
- Storage areas, including fruit cellars
- Old upholstered furniture
- Old newspapers, books
- Plants, soil and leaves
- Humidifiers, unless cleaned daily
- Old wallpaper
- Air conditioning systems left without cleaning
- Window sills

Pattern of Mold Allergy Symptoms

Increase in symptoms:

- Between 5 and 9PM, "cool evening air"
- In damp places (woods, leaky basements)
- Moving or raking leaves
- Sitting on the grass
- From September until the first heavy frost

Improvement of symptoms:

- In dry, clean areas
- When the temperature is below freezing and there is snow on the ground

CANDIDA ALBICANS

Candida, a yeast, is a pathogen that lives on mucous membranes and particularly in the colon of the gastrointestinal tract. There are about 140 different candida species, the majority being pathogenic, which under specific circumstances are able to cause candidiasis. Any internal organ can be involved in the disease process, as well as the skin and mucous membranes, depending upon the state of health of the individual (host resistance).

Concerns

- Candida creates toxins that weaken the immune system;
- According to European studies, the presence of any candida in the cultures of any body surface or organ is abnormal, even without manifestation of disease and should be prevented and treated vigorously.

FACTORS CONTRIBUTING TO CANDIDA INFECTION

- Broad-spectrum antibiotics (erythromycin, tetracycline, etc.), which kill friendly bacteria, providing more room for the candida to multiply;
- Sugar-rich and refined carbohydrate diets (yeast feeds on simple sugars);
- Birth control pills and pregnancy (hormonal changes promote yeast growth);
- Use of steroids in creams and tablets;
- Immunosuppressant treatments for cancer and use of cytostatic drugs (Imuran);
- Infancy and old age, when the immune system is either not yet fully developed or is beginning to be faulty;
- Genetically faulty immune system;
- Nutritional deficiencies;
- Starvation;
- Exposure to chemicals and subsequent alteration of immune defense;
- Indwelling catheters and invasive procedures (urinary catheters, central lines for parenteral nutrition);

INHALANTS

- Some disease states, e.g., diabetes, leukemia, cancer, high fever;
- Contact with other people in swimming pools or saunas;
- Sexual contact;
- Poor hygiene and overcrowding;

Chef Pierre

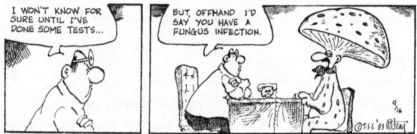

Typical Symptoms Caused by Candida

Any symptom from any organ or system can be caused by candida.

GENDER	SYMPTOM	
Men and Women	Fatigue	"Spacey" feeling
	Headache	Depression
	Numbness/tingling	Memory loss
	Abdominal pain	Bloating/gas
	Nasal congestion	Ear problems
	Muscle/joint pain	Skin problems
	Hives/itching	Athlete's foot
	Nail fungus	Constipation/diarrhea
Women	Vaginitis	Pelvic pain
	Vaginal discharge	Crying spells
	Menstrual problems	Infertility
	Decreased sex drive	PMS
Men	Prostatitis	Impotence
	Jock itch	

INHALANTS

Candida infection often causes an allergic response in the host individual that is infected.

Diagnosing Candida
- Discuss your case history with a doctor (one that is familiar with candida) and explore all predisposing factors;
- Yeast culture from vagina, mouth, sputum;
- Intradermal testing with candida extract to prove systemic reactions (symptoms), as well as to establish a dose of immunotherapy treatment;
- Blood test for candida.

(See page 229 in the Management section for ways to improve your health if you have excess candida.)

OUTDOOR INHALANTS

POLLENS
- Part of the reproduction system of plants;
- Although it is a seasonal occurrence, the wind can transport it thousands of miles (i.e., from the south during the middle of winter);
- It is at its highest in late evening and early morning, and is worse on dry/windy days.

Different pollens are tested in each environmental medicine office, depending on the geographical location.

INHALANTS

INHALANTS

The following pollens are common for Ontario:

TREE POLLENS		SEASON
Tree Mix #1 (early trees)	Sugar Maple, Tag Alder, White Ash, White Birch, American Elm, Common Cottonwood, Annual Wormwood	February to
Tree Mix #2 (late trees)	Hickory, Black Locust, Mulberry, Oak, Pine, Privet Willow, Poplar, Blue Spruce, Black Walnut	May

GRASS POLLENS	COMMON CONTACT	SEASON
Grass Mix #1		
Smooth Brome	cultivated for hay and pasture	May
Meadow Fescue	hay and pasture	to
Perennial Rye		
Timothy	waste places, hay, pasture	June
Grass Mix #2		
June	lawns, pastures	July
Quack	waste places	
Orchard		to
Red Top	lawns, pastures	
Sweet Vernal	fragrant meadow grass	September

WEED POLLENS	COMMON CONTACT	SEASON
WEED MIX • Weed Mix #1		
Cocklebur		August to September
Yellowdock (Curly Dock)		June to August
Burweed Marsh	waste places, where there	
Elder	has been water	
Goldenrod		August to September
Western Water Hemp		July to August
Lamb's Quarters		May to October

WEED POLLENS	COMMON CONTACT	SEASON
WEED MIX · Weed Mix #2		
Mugwort		July to October
Redrooted Pigweed		Late summer
English Plantain	lawn weed	April to September
Giant Ragweed	anywhere damp	August to September
Short Ragweed	roadsides	August to October
Russian Thistle (Tumbleweed)	June to September	
Sheep Sorrel (Field Sorrel)		May to June
Wormwood		

INHALANTS

PATTERN OF OUTDOOR INHALANT ALLERGY SYMPTOMS

Increase in symptoms:

- Outside, in season
- On a dry, sunny, windy day
- While mowing the lawn (grass and weed terpens)

Improvement of symptoms:

- Indoors with windows closed and/or air-conditioning
- After rain
- When season passes

CONCOMITANT AND SYNERGISTIC SENSITIVITIES

It is possible to be sensitive to a food only during certain inhalant seasons. This is what is referred to as a concomitant sensitivity. This differs from synergistic sensitivities. In this case, a reaction from one food is made worse by another. The following chart outlines some of the known concomitant and synergistic pairs.

PROVEN CONCOMITANT FOODS

When this is inhaled	And this is eaten = reaction
Ragweed	Milk, Mint
Iva Ciliata	Wheat
Sage	Potato
Pigweed	Pork
Grass	Legumes
Cedar	Beef, Yeasts
Elm	Milk, Mint
Cottonwood	Lettuce
Oak	Egg, Apple
Pecan	Corn, Banana
Mesquite	Cane Sugar, Orange
Dust	Oysters (seafood)

QUESTIONABLE CONCOMITANT FOODS

Dust	Nuts
Influenza vaccine	onion
Iva Ciliata	Tea
Chenopods	egg

PROVEN SYNERGISTIC FOODS

When this is eaten	Together with this = reaction
Corn	Banana
Beef	Yeasts
Cane Sugar	Orange
Milk	Mint
Egg	Apple

QUESTIONABLE SYNERGISTIC FOODS

Wheat	Tea
Pork	Chicken
Milk	Chocolate
Cola	Chocolate
Coffee	Cola–Chocolate

Source: D. W, Brown, Jr., M.D. Fredericksburg, Texas, 1/80

Chemicals

CHEMICALS

Chemicals are the building blocks of the world as we know it. The items we use in our daily life are composed of an array of chemical components. Our own bodies function through a complex set of chemical processes. It stands to reason, then, that chemicals that we breathe, eat, and touch interact with us. For some individuals, this interaction causes problems. The degree of sensitivity varies, and any substance can create difficulties. Of particular concern is the myriad of man-made and man-mobilized (naturally occurring and transformed by man) chemicals.

Since the advent of the chemical industry in the 1940s, thousands of chemicals have been produced and released into the air, water and food. Chemicals now contaminate even the remotest parts of the globe. Breast milk in Western countries is so dangerously contaminated that it would not pass FDA standards if it were a packaged product. In the Eastern seaboard and southwestern United States (the most highly industrialized parts), mothers are not recommended to breastfeed past six months, as the baby by then already has the maximum lifetime amounts of carcinogens in its cells. **When the food we eat is grown in nutrient-poor soil, watered with acid rain, sprayed with pesticides, and treated with food additives, and when the water we drink and the air we breathe are also contaminated, is it any wonder that chemicals have been detected in human blood and fat tissue?**

Research into toxic levels of some chemical exposures has occurred; however, the findings do not take all variables into consideration. Tests usually monitor the effects of one chemical in isolation, when in reality we are exposed to a wide variety. What are the interactive effects? Are the levels identified as safe for the average individual necessarily safe for the hypersensitive? What are the effects of long-term exposure? With these questions unanswered, we owe it to ourselves to increase our awareness of our chemical world.

Health Canada and the Ministry of the Environment are two government bodies that should be able to provide you with information about chemicals in your surrounding environment. Among the organizations that work for our benefit to fight the pollution from chemicals are the World Wildlife Fund and Pollution Probe.

Pollution Probe: 416-926–1907

www.pollutionprobe.org

World Wildlife Fund: 416-489–8800

www.wwf.ca

In the following pages, you will find key information pertaining to indoor and outdoor pollutants. Fact sheets on particularly troublesome chemicals have also been included. This material can be overwhelming, but remember, awareness is the first step towards positive action. With increased understanding comes the ability to control your exposure to chemicals and to improve your health. Refer to the Management section of this book for suggestions on how to do just that.

OUTDOOR POLLUTION

Outdoor pollution is a visible threat. In urban centers the "toilet bowl" ring of smog is plainly visible on the horizon. Further afield, lakes are devoid of life, maple trees are dying, the earth's protective ozone layer is threatened, and the list goes on. We are affected by pollution, and we, as individuals, also contribute to the problem. According to Pollution Probe, the largest class of toxic waste generators is Canadian households, with an average of forty-one litres a year per household. In addition, the average Canadian household throws away one ton of garbage per year. The following pages provide information regarding sources of outdoor pollution. Although many of the culprits are related to industry, don't forget you can make a difference in the quality of the air we breathe: become aware, be active, recycle, reuse, and look for safe alternatives to toxic products. Remember, changes begin in your own home.

FACTORS CONTRIBUTING TO OUTDOOR POLLUTION

It has recently been reported that toxic air triggers one thousand premature deaths and 5500 hospitalization per year in Toronto. When ozone is high, hospitalizations increase in Toronto by over 30%. Bad air promotes heart attacks, cardiovascular disease, asthma and lung cancer. It can contribute to any other disease in the susceptible individual. Pollution affects lung growth development and function in children. The effort of society should be to ensure that all children can spend at least part of their summer out of the city.

Your lungs are the gateway for life-giving oxygen to every cell in your body and unfortunately the gateway for toxins as well. Ventilate your lungs (and brain) with fresh air as often as possible. Going out of the city regularly, even for one or two days on a weekend into the countryside (but where it's not polluted with pesticides, e.g., orchard areas), can make a difference. The cleanest air is at sea level. I don't need a double blind study to prove there's a difference in my white cat's fur coat colour when she's at home in the city (yellowish) and after she's been at our cottage in the country for a couple of weeks (crystal white). The same thing will happen inside the body.

CHEMICALS

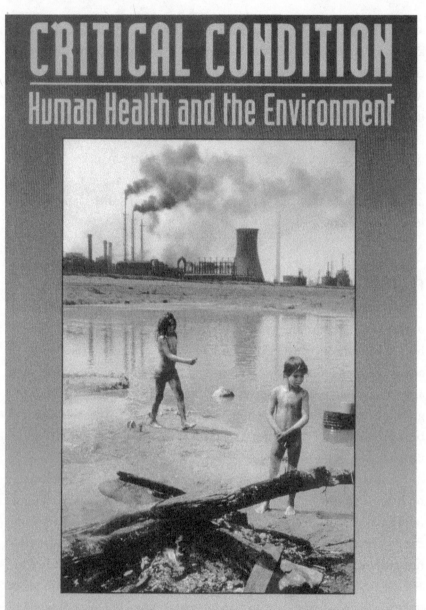

Critical Condition: Human Health and the Environment. *Edited by Eric Chivian, M.D. et al. The MIT Press, Cambridge, Mass. 1994. Photo: James Nachtwey, Magnum Photos, Inc.*

- Pesticides/herbicides from home lawns, orchards, golf courses, flower gardens, crops, parks
- Industry (metal, paper, rubber, oil refineries, smoke)
- Asphalt
- Engine exhaust (car, plane, diesel, lawn mowers, snowmobiles, etc.)
- Barbecues
- Burning fuel (paper, wood, garbage, oil, gas, coal and coal-burning electrical power plants)
- Paint
- Sewage fumes
- Chemicals leading to acid rain; SO_2, NO_2, and toxic rain; general volatile substances, PCBs, etc.

CHEMICALS

AIR QUALITY INDEX

In Ontario, the Ministry of the Environment and Environment Canada cooperatively deliver air quality advisories when widespread elevated air pollution levels are forecast.

They rely on two systems of measurement, the AQI and the API. The Air Quality Index (AQI) measures and reports on the six most common city air pollutants. The Air Pollution Index (API) is a sub-index of the AQI and its function is to warn of deteriorating air quality.

Automatic air monitoring stations are constantly analyzing the air, and their findings are reported to you in news and weather reports. During an advisory, people are encouraged to limit activities that contribute to pollution, such as reducing car usage, gas-powered lawn mowers, etc. Also, people with respiratory problems are advised to limit their outdoor activity. Smog alerts are triggered if air is poor or very poor.

The Ministry of the Environment provides AQI readings for your area, updated once a day:

www.ene.gov.on.ca

1-800-565-4923

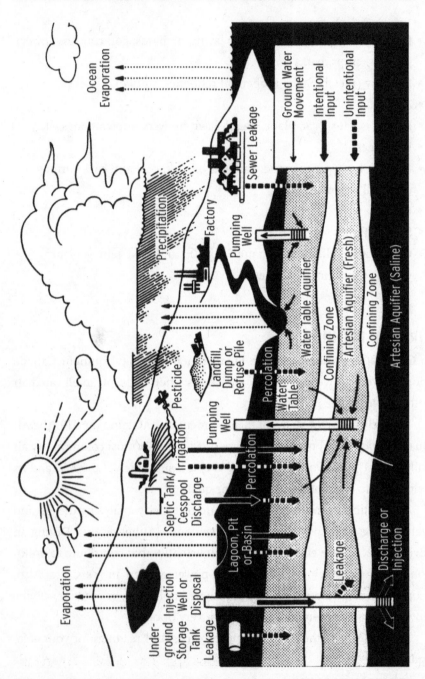

How waste-disposal practices can contaminate the groundwater system. Critical Condition: Human Health and the Environment. *Edited by Eric Chivion, M.D. et al. MIT Press, Cambridge, Mass. 1994.*

The following are the six most common city air pollutants contibuting to AQI:

CARBON MONOXIDE	CO	• Colourless, odourless, tasteless gas • Automobile emissions are primary source • First symptoms of CO poisoning are blurred vision and clumsiness (occurring at very high concentrations) • Lower concentrations can cause discomfort for people with heart or lung disease
NITROGEN DIOXIDE	NO_2	• Toxic, irritating gas • Emitted by all combustion processes, e.g., heating systems, cars, trucks • In combination with water, it can form acid rain • It helps form smog and acid aerosols (lung irritant) • Can irritate the lungs and lower resistance to respiratory infection
OZONE	O_3	• Colourless gas with a strong smell • Produced by the sun's photochemical action on hydrocarbons and nitrogen oxides • It is the biggest part of photochemical smog • Exposure to high concentrations of ozone results in chest tightness, coughing and wheezing • Responsible for agricultural crop loss in Ontario each year; causes noticeable leaf damage • More than 50% of Ontario's ozone comes from sources in the United States
SUSPENDED PARTICLES	SP	• Small particles of solid or liquid matter that stay suspended in the air in the form of dust, mist, aerosols, smoke, fumes, soot, etc. • Particles less than 10 microns can penetrate deep into the lungs and contribute to lung disease • Can also cause corrosion, material soiling, vegetation damage and visibility reduction
TOTAL REDUCED SULPHUR	TRS	• These are sulphur-containing compounds, such as hydrogen sulphide • Come from industrial sources such as pulp and paper mills, coke ovens and refineries • Also come from natural sources such as sulphur springs • Primary cause of odours (rotten egg smell) • Very high concentrations may cause nausea or headaches
SULPHUR DIOXIDE	SO_2	• Colourless gas that smells like burnt matches • Exposure to high concentrations can cause breathing discomfort, respiratory illness and aggravation of existing lung and heart disease • Damages leaves on trees and agricultural crops • Contributes to acid rain and helps form acid aerosols

CHEMICALS

Remember: ground-level ozone and the ozone layer in the stratosphere are not the same. Ozone 20 to 50 km above the earth's surface is naturally created and screens us from harmful ultraviolet radiation. Ground-level ozone is harmful to plants, animals and humans.

Source: Ministry of the Environment Fax-on-demand Publications
#063001 Ontario's Air Quality Index, Consumer Information

CHEMICALS

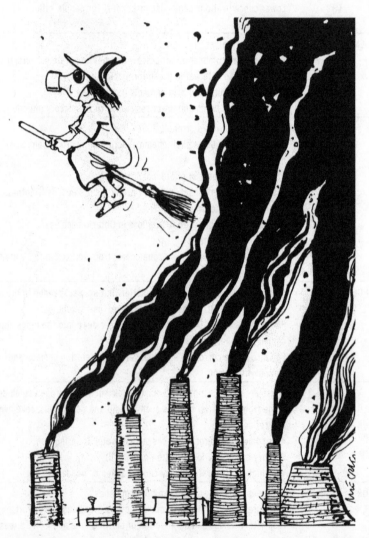

Artist: Andrzej Mleczko • Ekologia (or how to love nature) • Krakow Poland, 1991

Below is the **Air Quality Index** as provided by the Ministry of the Environment, Fax-on-demand publication service:

CATEGORY INDEX	0-15 VERY GOOD	16-31 GOOD	32-49 MODERATE	50-99 POOR	100+ VERY POOR
CO	No known harmful effects	No known harmful effects	Blood chemistry changes, but no noticeable impairment	Increasing symptoms in smokers with heart disease	Increasing symptoms in non-smokers with heart disease; blurred vision; some clumsiness
NO_2	No known harmful effects	Slight odour	Odour	Air smells and looks brown; some increase in bronchial reactivity in asthmatics	Increasing sensitivity for asthmatics and people with bronchitis
O_3	No known harmful effects	No known harmful effects	Respiratory irritation in sensitive people during vigorous exercise; people with heart/lung disorders at some risk; damages very sensitive plants	Sensitive people may experience irritation when breathing and possible lung damage when physically active; people with heart/lung disorders at greater risk; damage to some plants	Serious respiratory effects, even during light physical activity; people with heart/lung disorders at high risk; more vegetation damage
TRS	No known harmful effects	Slight odour	Odour	Strong odour	Severe odour; some people may experience nausea and headaches
SO_2 + SP	No known harmful effects	No known harmful effects	Damages vegetation (i.e., tomatoes, white beans) due to sulphur dioxide	Increased symptoms for people with chronic lung disease	Significant effects for asthmatics and people with bronchitis
SP	No known harmful effects	No known harmful effects	Some decrease in visibility	Decreased visibility; soiling evident	Increasing sensitivity for asthmatics and people with bronchitis
SO_2	No known harmful effects	Damages some vegetation in combination with ozone	Damages some vegetation	Odours; increasing vegetation damage	Increasing sensitivity for asthmatics and people with bronchitis

CHEMICALS

ACID RAIN

All volatile chemicals, gases SO_2 (sulphur dioxide) and NO_2 (nitrogen dioxide), as well as all pesticides and herbicides, are caught up in clouds and are transported thousands of kilometres from the polluted site. When the clouds release the accumulated moisture they have been carrying, the toxins are transported down to the earth with the rain and are soaked up in the soil. This acid rain depletes the soil of magnesium, the mineral required for effective functioning of chlorophyll in all green plants. Photosynthesis, the process whereby green plants absorb carbon dioxide and water and produce oxygen, cannot occur without chlorophyll and/or magnesium. Plants produce all of the earth's oxygen.

In very real terms, acid rain interferes with the production of oxygen necessary to sustain human life. An additional threat is presented by acid rain in respect to heavy metals. As minerals such as calcium and magnesium are removed from the soil, less nutrient-dense foods are grown and naturally present heavy metals leach out of the soil and enter into our foods. Plants and foods containing a lower level of magnesium are more susceptible to mold overgrowth and mycotoxin contamination.

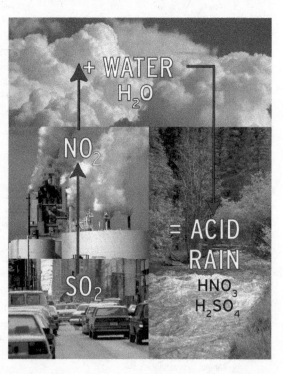

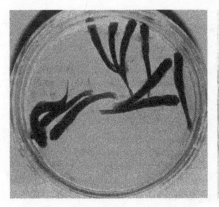
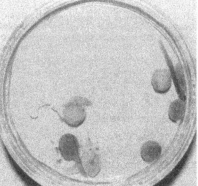

Fish fry in water with a normal pH.

Fish fry in water with a low pH caused by acid rain. When the pH of a water body goes below a certain level, fish fry either die or, if they survive, are hatched with severe deformities. Source: Environment Canada 1982

CHEMICALS

OZONE (O₃)

Facts

Naturally occurring:

- highest concentration in the upper atmosphere, 10–50 km in altitude
- this ozone layer absorbs most of the ultraviolet light coming to earth
- Produced through photochemical action of the sun on hydrocarbons or through electrical storms

Man-made:

- pungent, colourless gas
- can be very bothersome even in small amounts (.04ppm)
- individuals with respiratory difficulty are particularly bothered by ozone

Major Source

- Created by electrical equipment such as kitchen appliance motors, sewing machines and power tool motors;

- Electrostatic air cleaners, ion generators, photocopiers, and computers and computer printers;
- Present during smog conditions, electrical storms and near power transmission lines.

OZONE HOLES

Man-made pollution emits a lot of chlorine into the atmosphere in the form of chlorofluorocarbons, discharged from air-cooling systems, plastic foam production, propellants used in spray cans, auto exhaust, etc. This chlorine reacts with the ozone in the upper atmosphere (10 to 60 km above) causing ozone to disappear, thus creating huge holes in the ozone layer. This reduces the protectiveness of the ozone layer, allowing an excess of UV light to reach the earth. This has a detrimental effect on the food chain in the animal and plant kingdom by killing plankton, a major food source. It also causes increased incidents of skin cancer.

Depending on various conditions, a different amount of UV light can reach the earth daily; therefore, a UV Index was created.

UV-B Degree of Danger Scale:

UV-B is measured on a scale of 0 to 10, with 10 being a typical amount you would receive on a summer day in the tropics—where UV-B is at its highest on earth. The higher the number on the UV index, the more UV-B you will get, and the faster you'll sunburn.

What does the UV index mean to me?

UV INDEX	CATEGORY	SUNBURN TIME
over 9	extreme	less than 15 minutes
7-9	high	about 20 minutes
4-7	moderate	about 30 minutes
0-4	low	more than one hour

CHEMICALS

When the UV index is over 9, UV-B is extremely strong, and you will burn in less than 15 minutes. (Sunburn times are for light untanned skin, the times would be somewhat longer for those with darker skin.)

The major concern with UV light is development of skin cancer. The higher the UV index, the higher the risk for cancer.

Sunscreens do not necessarily protect or shield the skin from UV light. Rather, a good level of vitamins A, C, E and other anti-oxidants would be beneficial in helping protect the skin from developing cancer.

UV LIGHT

UV light depletes nutrient content in all plants (fruit, vegetable, grain) [see Organic Foods section page 149]. This is due to the effect of UV light on the beneficial microorganism, **mycorrhizza**, a fungus which lives in the colony or web around plant roots. Its role is to deliver nutrients from the soil to the plant roots, and in return the roots deliver "sweets" from photosynthesis to feed the fungus. 80% of the world's plants, including crops and forests, thrive because of the friendly relationship between plants and this fungus. They are connected underground, which allows the fungus to provide plants with water and nutrients. It can also extract nutrients that plants usually can't use e.g., protein from dead organisms.

UV light stresses the fungus, which then stores the nutrients instead of delivering them to the roots. This encourages parasites, pathogens and disease microbes to attack the fungi to get at its nutrients. Unfriendly organisms increase in the soil. Plants weakened by poor nutrient levels are more vulnerable to attack by malevolent pathogens. The cycle of using pesticides usually starts at this point.

Plants protect their leaves from UV light, which in excess can kill them, by manufacturing bioflavinoids. To do this, they need nitrogen delivered by the friendly fungus which is already compromised, needs nitrogen for its own survival and doesn't deliver enough to the plant.

http://mycorrhiza.ag.utk.edu/

ORGANOCHLORINES

Facts

- organic chemicals containing hydrogen and carbon plus chlorine (also called, chlorinated hydrocarbons)
- almost all are toxic and carcinogenic
- they accumulate in body fats, where they can be released into the blood
- stated safe levels: PVC and PCB are hazardous at any level and .01ppm of organochlorines in foods is a definite risk. Solvents at a level of 100 to 500ppm are also a serious risk.
- Canadian and US household products are labelled as hazardous, and ingredients are listed. The identifying word for this group of chemicals is "chloro." Any numbers indicate the chemical structure.
- difficult to remove from the environment (persistent organic pollutants —POPs)

Major Sources of Exposure

- liquid solvents: cleaning products, dry cleaning fluids, paints
- some stabilized plastics: PVC, PCB
- pesticides: most toxic and persistent of the group
- chloroform gas
- in foods
- wood preservatives
- industrial emissions
- chlorine in water

PCBs—POLYCHLORINATED BIPHENYLS

Facts
- chemically very stable; they cannot be broken down, therefore there is no way of getting rid of them
- volatile, therefore they travel as a gas and through water
- insoluble in water
- concentrate in fats
- can be inhaled, swallowed, and absorbed through skin
- most are stored in Smithville, by Ontario Hydro

Major Sources of Exposure
- before the 1970s they were widely used in many products, after 1979 their use in new products was banned; tons remain in storage
- carbonless copy paper, fish, cooling fluid used in transformers

VOLATILE ORGANIC COMPOUNDS, VOCs

Examples
Alkanes, alkenes, naphthas, benzenes, toluene, xylene, ethers, mineral spirits, alcohols (methyl, ethyl), ketones, aldehydes, propane, butane, polymers, monomers, trichloroethane, trichloroethylene, tetrachloroethylene

Form
- liquid at room temperature

Facts
- contain hydrogen and carbon plus chlorine
- base of many synthetic substances

CHEMICALS

- readily evaporated, particularly with the addition of heat
- can be explosive
- can be extracted from petroleum (oil, gas) or produced synthetically
- high concentrations are reached very easily
- some of these accumulate in body fat

Major Sources of Exposure

- in foods, in water
- added to solids, i.e., plastic
- paint
- cleaning solvents
- wax, polish
- gasoline, oil, natural gas, propane, butane
- dry-cleaning fluids
- artificial and natural scents, perfumes

CHEMICALS

Toluene:	solvent-based adhesives, paints, waxes, cleaners, upholstery, plastic
Napthalene:	mothballs, moth-proofed fabrics
Benzene:	felt-tipped markers, varnishes, solvents, paints, mothballs, used in the production of nylon, anthraquinone dyes (toxic above 1 ppm) can cause drunken behaviour, lightheadedness, disorientation, fatigue, loss of appetite, and cancer

Organochlorines, volatile organic compounds, as well as chlorinated pesticides can be measured both in the blood as well as in fat biopsies of individuals exposed to them. A large majority of these chemicals are carcinogenic.

Common Exposure Sources of Volatile Organic Compounds (Solvents)

Volatile organic solvents	Fuel & exhaust	Paint, ink glue	Synthetic textiles, plastics	Drinking water	Soil, grain, building fumigant	Industrial degreaser & solvent
Benzene	X	M	M	X		
Toluene	X	X		X		X
Ethyl-benzene	X	M	M	X		
Xylene	X	X	M	X		X
Styrene	X		M	X		
Trimethyl-benzene	X	M	M	X		X
Dichloro-methane		X		X		X
Trichloro-ethane			X	X		X
Trichloro-ethylene		X	X	X		X
Tetrachloro-ethylene				X	X	X
Dichloro-benzene				X	X	

X, present in final product; M, used in manufacturing process.

CHEMICALS

Common Exposure Sources of Volatile Organic Compounds (Solvents) cont'd

Volatile organic solvents	Refrigerant impurity	Dry cleaning solvents	Detergents	Pharma-ceuticals	Gasoline additive	Insecti-cides
Benzene			M	M	M	
Toluene		X			X	X
Ethyl-benzene					X	
Xylene		X			X	X
Styrene						
Trimethyl-benzene					X	
Dichloro-methane	X					
Trichloro-ethane		X				
Trichloro-ethylene	X	X				
Tetrachloro-ethylene		X		M		
Dichloro-benzene						X

X, present in final product; M, used in manufacturing process.

Adapted from J. Laseter, Accu-Chem Laboratories, Inc.

PESTICIDES, HERBICIDES AND FUNGICIDES

Pesticides accumulate in body fat and can be released into the blood stream. An "EPA study of random blood samples from 54 locations revealed 99% carry at least detectable levels of the pesticide DDT." In addition, "a four year National Health and Nutrition Examination survey showed pentachlorophenol—a wood preservative that carries dioxin—in nearly 80% of urine specimens collected nationwide." Further discussion of these chemicals will be found in the "Special Interest" section featured in Hormone Disrupting Chemicals on page 270.

M. Brown, Laying Waste: The Poisoning of America by Toxic Chemicals, New York, 1979

Most pesticides fall into three categories:

Chlorinated Hydrocarbons

D.D.T.	dieldrin	P.C.B.
Lindane (BHC)	aldrin	P.C.P.
Endrin	chlordane	P.B.B.
T.C.D.D.	mirex	heptachlor

Organophosphates,* some of the most deadly being:

Phosdrin	diazinon	ethion
Parathion	ethyl-parathion	dursban
Mevinphos	methyl-parathion	Roundup™
Malathion	tetraethylhydrophosphate	

Phenoxy Acid Herbicide

2,4,5T	2,4,5T methyl ester
Silvex	silvex methyl ester
Silvex	silvex iso-octyl ester
2,4-D	2,4-DB

Note: Agent Orange is a combination of 2,4-D and 2,4,5-T.

Organophosphates paralyze the parasympathetic nervous system by inhibiting cholinesterase (the enzyme metabolizing the neurotransmitter, acetylcholine). The parasympathetic nervous system is a component of the entire autonomic nervous system and supplies nerves to every single organ, therefore, symptoms from any part of the body due to organophosphate exposure can be manifested.

Common Contacts with Pesticides:

- Household pesticides, such as dieldrin, dissipate into the air we breathe;
  - "No Pest" strips, insect sprays or coils, mothballs
  - moth repellent may also be present in dry-cleaned articles or moth-proofed blankets and rugs
- Exterminator treatments
- Home foundations (insecticides deter bugs)
- The foods we eat are sprayed during growth, shipping, storage—the chemicals used saturate the plant cells, therefore, they cannot be washed off and peeling doesn't do a complete job (e.g., during their growth cycle apples are sprayed seventeen times). Vegetables and fruit in supermarkets usually contain nine or more pesticides.
- Imported fabrics are often fumigated upon entry into the country
- Pesticides and herbicides are used in both urban and rural settings
- Garden products, some combination "weed and feed" products
- Some parks, all golf courses, are heavily sprayed with pesticides and herbicides
- Majority of home lawns use herbicides
- Road sides, railway sides, are routinely sprayed
- Aerial spraying of cities—mosquito—Winnipeg, Vancouver, entire coast of South USA 1999
- Wood preservative (a dioxin—highly toxic; a sealer must be used over top of the chemical treatment)
- Some paints and varnishes contain pesticides
- The majority of public institutions (hotels, schools, nursing homes, hospitals, restaurants, etc.) are sprayed at least twice per year. Kitchens

in these institutions are sprayed every six weeks.

All pesticides contain solvents to aid in the penetration of the poison into the target organism. These solvents are not listed as part of the ingredients, as they are termed "inert ingredients."

In a survey of 6800 patients suffering from environmental exposures, 80% knew the time, place and circumstances under which they became ill. From this group, 60% knew that the cause of their illness was exposure to pesticides.

Ashford, N., Miller C. *Chemical Exposures, Low Level, High States.* Van Nostrand Reinhold, 1991, pg. 5.

Common Contacts with Fungicides:

- Tobacco
- Packing boxes
- Grocery store items
- Wall paper paste
- Rubber
- Wool products
- Sprayed crops

PETROCHEMICALS

Petroleum

- A natural product found within the earth. It is produced over time, through the chemical restructuring of crushed organic materials. In simple terms, it is a chain of carbons.
- Other chemical structures are also created during the formation of petroleum.
- Petroleum forms the basis of many synthetic chemicals, i.e., phenol, ethanol, benzyl alcohol, formaldehyde, plastics, glycols.

Major Sources of Exposure

- mineral oil
- fuels; oil, kerosene, gasoline, and car exhaust, old car parts, lubricating oil
- paint
- kerosene
- compressed gas in propellant spray cans
- wax candles (paraffin)
- nylon fabrics and carpet
- rubber carpet underpads
- food preservatives; BHA (butylated hydroxyanisole), BHT (butylated hydroxytoluene)
- Pesticides, herbicides, fungicides, wood preservatives

Pyridine (C_5H_5N):

- toxic and water soluble flammable liquid
- a by-product of cooking
- can occur naturally
- it is the parent of many naturally occurring organic compounds
- used as a solvent and in pharmacological drugs used as a waterproofing agent

Pyrol (C_4H_5N)

- toxic liquid
- a parent of many biologically important substances
- exists in the body, i.e., in bile pigment

Tiophene (C_4H_4S)

- from coal tar
- resembles benzene

HYDROCARBONS
- The basic building blocks of life
- Refers to all chemical structures containing hydrogen and carbon
- Chemicals that fall into this category can be natural (sugars), or synthetic (DDT); in either case they are considered to be organic (**Note:** organic chemicals also include those with a carbon/oxygen or carbon/hydrogen/oxygen chain)

FORMALDEHYDE

Facts
- commonly called formalin
- gas (highly active), or liquid
- a hydrocarbon
- an industrial chemical manufactured from methanol/natural gas and some lower petroleum hydrocarbons
- according to Rousseau, there is no safety threshold level; the Canadian government has set a level at 0.1ppm; this is the same level at which the smell is detectable; it is a carcinogen
- 1 out of 5 individuals are sensitive to formaldehyde, and it is often a factor in the onset of chemical hypersensitivity
- can aggravate minor illnesses and trigger others

Major Sources
- **Building materials:**
    - urea formaldehyde resins in insulation, particleboard and plywood are the biggest problem. They evaporate slowly and remain active for months/years. In fabrics the process is even slower;
    - resin glues, plastics, foams, insulation of homes and mobile homes;
    - additive in plaster, concrete and other related products that are impermeable to liquids;

CHEMICALS

– component of; plywood, particleboard, wallboard, wood preservative, chipboard, resins, wood veneer, latex paints, enamels.

- **Preservative, fungicide, stabilizer, germicide:**
  – polishes, waxes, adhesives, fats and oils, rodent and insect poison,
  detergent soaps, hair setting, hair shampoo and spray, photographic products, cosmetics, US maple syrup, milk, disinfectant in
  the fermentation industry, cleaning of surgical instruments, manufacturing of antibiotics, hospital mouthwashes and antiperspirants,
  embalming fluids (along with alcohol, glycerol, phenol), tooth-
  paste, disinfectants, cleaning supplies, contraceptive creams, air
  deodorizers.

- **Fabric treatment:**
  – wash and wear, permanent press, anti-wrinkle, anti-static, stiffening
  on lightweight knits, chlorine-resistant finishes, moth-proof
  finishes, mildew-resistant fabrics, suede and chamois, fireproofing,
  dye industry; improve stability, stripping agents, dyes, tanning of
  leather, increase absorbency of paper products including feminine
  hygiene items, facial tissue, dry cleaning (see Fabrics section,
  page 130)

- **Combustion:**
  – cigarette smoke, burning fuel, incinerated waste materials,
  incomplete combustion of hydrocarbons in gas and diesel engines

- **Miscellaneous:**
  – intermediate in the synthesis of alcohols, acids, explosives
  – deodorizer in industrial and public places
  – used in the manufacture of synthetic vitamins A and E
  – mildew preventative in fruits and vegetables
  – preservative and coagulant of rubber latex
  – toxoids and vaccines
  – newsprint, printing-etching materials, inks (marking)
  – nailpolish and fingernail hardeners, wavesets and fixatives
  – foam pillows, orthopedic casts, kidney dialysis units
  – used in photography (darkroom developing)

ALCOHOLS

Facts
- a class name for a group of chemicals all containing one or more carbinol groups
- can be created from grains and sugars, or synthesized from petroleum

Forms

Ethyl Alcohol: See the following page

Amyl Alcohol: From ethyl alcohol; used as a solvent

Isopropyl: Used to manufacture antifreeze, rubbing alcohol and solvents

Methyl Alcohol: Also known as methanol; poisonous, used in antifreeze

Glycerol: Used for sweetening and preserving food; also used in cosmetics, perfumes, inks, and some glues/cements

Menthol: It is an alcohol obtained from diverse mint oils or prepared synthetically. Used in perfumes, used as a flavouring. Found in cold and nasal medications because of the cooling effect on nasal passages.

Butylalcohol

Ethylene glycol: antifreeze

Glycerin: adhesives, aftershave lotions, antifreeze, astringents, cosmetics (particularly caked or compact), cough drops, disinfectants, dry cleaning agents, eye drops, fabric, fabric softeners, face masks, fire retardant for fabrics, flavourings, floor polishes, food additives, freckle lotion, furniture polish, inks, latex paints, leather, liquid soaps, margarines, modeling clay, mouthwashes, nail polish, oven cleaners, paper, perfume, pharmaceuticals, plastics, polishes, polyurethane foam, shortening, solvent, styptic pencils, suntan preparations, tobacco, toothpastes, window cleaners.

CHEMICALS

CHEMICALS

FOOD CONSTITUENTS OF ALCOHOLIC BEVERAGES

	Corn	Malt	Rye	Wheat	Oats	Rice	Potato	Grape	Plum	Citrus	Apple	Pear	Apricot	Peach	Cherry	Berries	Honey	Juniper	Coconut	Taro	Cactus	Beet	Cane	Yeast
Whiskey																								
Straight Corn	X	X	+	+	+	+																X	X	X
Straight Bourbon	X	X	X	+	+	+																X	X	X
Straight Malt	X	X	X	+	+	+																X	X	X
Straight Rye	X	X	X	+	+	+																X	X	X
Straight Wheat	X	X	+	X	+	+																+	X	X
Blended Straight	X	X	X	X	+	+																X	X	X
Blended Straight Corn	X	X	X	X	X	X																X	X	X
Blended Straight Bourbon	X	X	X	X	X	X																X	X	X
Blended Straight Malt	X	X	X	X	X	X																X	X	X
Blended Straight Rye	X	X	X	X	X	X																X	X	X
Blended Straight Rye-Malt	X	X	X	X	X	X																X	X	X
Blended Straight Wheat	X	X	X	X	X	X																X	X	X
Blended	X	X	X	X	X	X		X	X	X	X											X	X	X
Spirit	X	X	X	X	X	X		X	X	X	X											X	X	X
Canadian	X	X	X	X				X	X														X	X
Blended Canadian	X	X	X	X	X	X		X	X	X												X	X	X
Unblended Scotch		X	X																				X	X
Scotch	X	X	+	+	+	+	X																X	X
Blended Scotch	X	X	+	+	+	+		X	X	X													X	X
Blended Scotch Type	X	X	X	X	X	X		X	X	X												X	X	X
Irish		X	X	X	X																		X	X
Blended Irish	X	X	X	X	X			X	X	X													X	X
Blended Irish Type	X	X	X	X	X	X		X	X	X												X	X	X
Malt Beverages																								
Beer	X	X	+	+	+	X																+	+	X
Ale	X	X	+	+	+	X																+	+	X
Gin																								
Grain Spirits	X	X	X	+	+	+												X						X
Cane Spirits																		X					X	X
Vodka																								
Domestic	X	X	X	X	+	+	+	+	+	+	+	+	+	+	+	+	+	+	+	+	+	+	+	X
Some Imports					X																	X		
Rum																								
Domestic								X															X	X
Jamaican																							X	X
Misc.																								
Aquavit							X											X						X
Arak						X																	X	X
Sake						X																		X
Tequila	?																				X			X
Okolehao																				X			X	X

X=indicates most commonly employed source material

+=indicates permitted material used in relatively smaller amounts, less frequently or at times of shortages

FOOD CONSTITUENTS OF ALCOHOLIC BEVERAGES

	Corn	Barley-Rye-Wheat	Oats	Rice	Potato	Grape	Plum	Citrus	Apple	Pear	Apricot	Peach	Cherry	Berries	Juniper	Coconut	Cinamon	Chocolate	Mint	Misc. Herbs	Honey	Beet	Cane	Yeast	Water
Brandy																									
Grape	+					X																+	+	X	X
Raisin	+					X																+	+	X	X
Cognac						X																+	+	X	X
Plum							X															+	+	X	X
Applejack	+								X													+	+	X	X
Apricot	+										X											+	+	X	X
Peach	+											X										+	+	X	X
Cherry	+												X									+	+	X	X
Blackberry	+													X								+	+	X	X
Fruit	+					X	X	X	X	X	X	X	X	X								+	+	X	X
Neutral	+					X	X	X	X	X	X	X	X	X								+	+	X	X
Juniper															X							?	?	X	X
Fruit Flavored Brandy	X	X	+	+	+	X	X	X	X	X	X	X	X	X		+	X	X	X	X	+	X	X	X	X
Cordials and Liquers	X	X	+	+	+	X	X	X	X	X	X	X	X	X		+	X	X	X	X	+	X	X	X	X
Wine																									
Grape	X				+	X																X	X	X	X
Raisin	X					X																X	X	X	X
Sherry	X				X	X																X	X	X	X
Champagne					X	X																X		X	X
Plum	X						X															X	X	X	X
Prune	X						X															X	X	X	X
Citrus	X							X														X	X	X	X
Cider	X								X													X	X	X	X
Perry	X									X												X	X	X	X
Apricot	X										X											X	X	X	X
Peach	X											X										X	X	X	X
Cherry	X												X									X	X	X	X
Blackberry	X													X								X	X	X	X
Raspberry	X													X								X	X	X	X
Fruit	X					X	X	X	X	X	X	X	X	X							X	X	X	X	X
Honey	X																					X	X	X	X
Flavoured	X					X	X	X	X	X	X	X	X	X						X		X	X	X	X
Vermouth	+	+	+			X														X		X	X	X	X

Source: Randolph, Theron G., *Environmental Medicine—Beginnings and Bibliographies of Clinical Ecology* pg. 185 ISBN: 0-943771-01-3, 1987

CHEMICALS

ETHANOL/ETHYL ALCOHOL

SYNTHETIC

Facts
- commonly called synthetic ethyl alcohol, S.E.A.
- one of a group of chemicals known as alcohols
- made from ethylene gas by oil companies

Major Sources
- Toiletry and drug preparations such as perfumes, aftershave, and other scented products, deodorant, soaps, shampoo, hair spray, cosmetics;
- Used in the production of rubber;
- It is a solvent for various hydrocarbons present in crude petroleum, therefore, it is found in petroleum and its derivatives, i.e., asphalt;
- Used to make ether and to sterilize surgical instruments;
- Disinfectants, rubbing alcohol;
- Flavouring extracts;
- Shellac, paints, varnish;
- Glue;
- A by-product of combustion (automobiles, heating systems), present in smog;
- Insect sprays, mothballs;
- Detergents;
- Ripening of bananas, gas roasting of coffee, processing of beef, cane, and corn sugars;

NATURAL

Facts
- A sensitivity to natural alcohol usually indicates intolerance to the product used for fermentation, e.g., brewer's yeast, rather than the alcohol itself.

Major Sources

- A product of the fermentation of grain, corn, potato, artichokes, sugar beets, sweet fruit, and cane sugar (see chart on pp. 100-101).

PHENOL (SYNTHETIC)

Facts

- commonly called carbolic acid, hydroxybenzene
- a group of chemicals within the alcohol nomenclature, including: biphenyl, pentachlorophenol (PCP), cresol (methylphenol)
- a derivative of coal tar/petroleum
- easily detected odour
- in hypersensitive people reactions have been noted at .002ppm [1]

Major Sources

- Household cleaners: Pinesol, Lysol; mildew products; wax; shoe polish; metal polishes; laundry starches; synthetic detergents (including dishwasher detergents);
- Used as an antiseptic;
- Used as a preservative;
- Medications; some allergy antigen extracts, nasal sprays, bronchial mists, cough syrups, eye drops, antihistamines, cold capsules, decongestants, first aid ointments, aspirin, acne medication;
- jute and hemp fibre products; carpet backing, area rugs, rope, twine;
- cosmetics; e.g., mascara, liquid eyeliner, cream rouges and shadows
- Hair care products; hairspray, setting lotion, shampoo, colouring;
- Phenolic resin;
- Lining in some canned goods;
- In combination with formaldehyde to create bakelite (found in telephone parts, children's toys, refrigerator storage trays, thermal insulation);
- In pesticides and herbicides, germicidal paints;
- In wood and coal tar;

CHEMICALS

- In tobacco smoke;
- Synthetic fibres and flame retardant finishes;
- Some building materials, including: adhesives, epoxy, enamel paint, fibreglass, insulation (thermal and acoustical), plywood, sealants, solvents, wood preservative;
- Miscellaneous: photographic solutions, food additives, explosives, dyes, perfumes, polyurethane and plastics, paints (poster, tempera, watercolour), shaving cream, matches, inks (drawing, printer's, stamp pad)

NATURALLY OCCURRING PHENOLS

Phenolics occur in foods we eat and in many natural objects in the world around us. For example, they are a toxic element in poison ivy and poison oak and are present in thyme oil (used in the production of menthol). They can also occur in spring water due to humus or natural coal in or around the spring. Unfortunately, some individuals react to these natural preservatives. In such cases, symptoms are experienced from a wide range of foods. **Treatment of phenolic sensitivity with sublingual drops often improves tolerance to foods and inhalants.** The following list indicates the presence of thirty-one phenolics in a variety of foods.

Source: Ber Abram, M.D., F.R.C.P. (C). "Neutralization of Phenolic (Aromatic) Food Compounds in a Holistic General Practice." The Journal of Orthomolecular Psychiatry Fourth Quarter 1983—Volume 12, Number 4. pp. 283-291

CHEMICALS

PHENOLIC (AROMATIC) FOOD COMPOUNDS

TABLE I — CHEMICALS

ALLERGENS IN FOODS!
by Robert Gardner PhD. Brigham Young University

ALLERGENS	Caffeine	Camphor	Capsaicin	Cinnamaldehyde	Cinnamic Acid	Coumarin/Scopoletin	Eugenol	Folic Acid	Gallic Acid	Indole	Isoascorbic Acid	Malvin (Anthocyanidins)	Menadione (Napthoquinones)	Nacin	Nicotine	Phenylalanine	Phenyl (Benzyl) Isothoicyanate	Phlorizin or Phloridzin	Piperine	Piperonal	Riboflavin	Rutin-Quercetin (Flavonol)	Saccarub	Thymine	Thymol	Uric Acid	Vanillin	Vanillylamine	Vitamin C	Vitamin E	Apiol
Allspice									•																						
Almond							•		•												•								•		•
Anise						•																									•
Apple				•	•				•			•	•						•			•					•				
Apricot				•					•												•	•					•				
Avocado				•					•			•	•									•					•				
Banana				•	•				•			•	•		•		•			•		•					•				
Barley					•				•			•										•									
Bean, kidney												•						•	•			•									
Bean, string												•						•	•			•									
Beef				•	•										•		•	•	•	•		•					•		•		•
Beet							•		•	•			•							•		•									
Beet sugar				•					•									•	•	•		•									
BHR/BHT				•					•																						
Blueberry				•					•			•																			
Blue food color*				•					•																						
Brocolli																	•					•									
Buckwheat																						•							•		
Cabbage				•					•			•					•					•									
Calif. Bay Laurel						•																									•
Cane sugar				•					•													•									
Cantaloupe									•												•								•		
Carrot				•	•	•			•								•					•									•
Cashew									•						•		•				•	•							•		
Celery				•	•	•	•					•	•									•									•
Cheese				•	•	•	•											•	•			•							•	•	
Cherry									•			•	•								•	•					•				
Chicken					•							•					•		•			•									
Cinnamon			•	•	•		•														•	•					•				
Cloves				•			•		•			•															•		•		•
Cocoa/chocolate	•			•	•		•						•				•					•					•				
Corn				•					•			•										•								•	
Cream of Tartar									•																						
Cucumber									•												•	•									
Dill						•																								•	
Egg				•					•			•	•					•		•		•									
Garlic																		•		•									•		
Gelatin																				•		•							•		
Ginger																															
Grape				•								•	•					•		•		•							•		
Halibut				•					•									•		•											
Honey, clover																				•	•										
Honeydew melon																															
Lamb					•							•					•	•	•	•		•							•		
Lemon				•	•	•			•													•					•		•	•	
Lettuce				•	•				•			•	•					•		•		•				•	•		•		
Lime						•																									
Mace						•																								•	
Malt																					•								•		
Mango								•																							

PHENOLIC (AROMATIC) FOOD COMPOUNDS

TABLE I (cont.) CHEMICALS

ALLERGENS IN FOODS!

by
Robert Gardner PhD.
Brigham Young University

Food	Caffeine	Camphor	Capsaicin	Cinnamaldehyde	Cinnamic Acid	Coumarin/Scopoletin	Eugenol	Folic Acid	Gallic Acid	Indole	Isoascorbic Acid	Malvin (Anthocyanidins)	Menadione (Napthoquinones)	Nacin	Nicotine	Phenylalanine	Phenyl (Benzyl) Isothoicyanate	Phlorizin or Phloridzin	Piperine	Piperonal	Riboflavin	Rutin-Quercetin (Flavonol)	Saccarub	Thymine	Thymol	Uric Acid	Vanillin	Vanillylamine	Vitamin C	Vitamin E	Apiol
Maple syrup									•																						
Milk (cow)			•		•		•		•		•					•	•		•	•	•	•							•		•
Milk (human)													•														•	•			
Mints																									•						
Mustard																•	•														
Nectarine																	•														
Nutmeg						•			•		•								•										•		•
Okra									•											•											
Onion			•	•					•			•	•			•				•		•							•		
Orange				•	•	•			•										•			•							•		•
Parsnips			•						•										•			•									
Peach									•											•		•									
Pear									•			•								•		•									
Pea			•	•	•				•	•	•					•			•			•									•
Peanut																•			•										•		
Pecan									•		•																		•		
Pepper, black			•	•					•							•			•	•		•									•
Pineapple			•						•		•									•		•									
Pork																				•		•									
Potato			•		•				•						•					•		•							•		
Pumpkin									•											•											
Rabbit																				•											
Radish									•		•						•														
Raspberry									•			•	•									•									
Red food color*									•																						
Rice				•																		•				•					
Sage																															
Salmon											•								•			•									
Sassafras					•																									•	
Soybean				•	•				•							•	•		•			•							•	•	
Spinach									•																						
Squash									•			•								•		•		•							
Strawberry				•						•	•	•	•									•							•		
Sweet potato																			•			•									
Tapioca			•	•																		•				•					
Thyme																															
Tomato			•	•	•	•			•	•	•				•	•			•	•		•							•	•	
Trout				•																		•		•	•						
Tuna				•							•								•	•											
Turkey				•							•									•											
Vanillin/vanilla									•											•		•									
Venison																			•	•							•				
Walnut						•			•		•																			•	
Watermelon									•		•										•	•									
Wheat				•					•													•									
Yam									•													•	•								
Yeast				•											•				•	•	•	•							•		
Yellow food color*									•																						

ASBESTOS

Facts

- a group of naturally occurring silicate minerals that separate into thin, strong fibres which are heat-resistant and durable
- upon deterioration, tends to break down into a dust of microscopic size fibres, at which point it becomes dangerous
- easily penetrates body through inhalation or ingestion
- no safe level of exposure
- fibres can remain in the body for many years
- causes pulmonary fibrosis, pleural calcification, pleural mesothelioma, cancer
- known symptoms generally do not appear for 10–30 years after the exposure
- smokers at higher risk of developing asbestos-related diseases
- widely used until the 1970s—professional advice needed for safe removal
- asbestos fibres have been found in lungs and other tissues of the general population, especially urban dwellers

Major Sources of Exposure

- Construction, industry, mining, shipbuilding;
- Older homes and products: textured paint, patching compounds, insulation, acoustical tiles, pipe blankets, pipe tape, vinyl flooring, stove pads;
- Currently still used in thousands of products, including roof shingles, building panels, water and sewer pipes, roof coatings, floor tiles, electrical insulating materials, specialized thermal insulation, elevator brakes, and protective aprons and gloves, brake pads and linings, clutch facings, gaskets;

CHEMICALS

CHEMICALS

RADON

Facts
- colourless, odourless gas
- this is a natural chemical resulting from the radioactive decay in radium
- it occurs in certain geological zones (e.g., Southern Ontario, Quebec, N.Y. State, Colorado, Pennsylvania)
- as the radon breaks down, even more hazardous substances attach themselves to dust and are inhaled; the radiation is then released within the lungs
- the allowed level of exposure in the US is 4pCi/L, but there can be effects at 1pCi/L
- building contamination depends upon paths of entry, and the direction of air flowing through these paths

Major Sources
- Soils, building materials (i.e. stone, cement), ground water in key geological zones
- Also encountered in uranium and phosphate mining

General Radon Inquiries
- In Canada, contact the following: Health Protection Branch; Food, Drugs, Cosmetics, Radiation and Medical Devices, 2301 Midland Ave., 416-973-1600. For other areas, make local inquiries.

For testing information:
Check your local phone book under Engineers/Environmental

HEAVY METALS

These metals occur naturally. They are present in our food, water and air. They accumulate in our body from ingestion or from absorption through the skin. They are difficult to get rid of. They can be analyzed in an individual's blood or tissue. Hair analysis can be very useful in assessing heavy metal exposure and intoxication. 24-hour urine challenge tests assess levels of heavy metals, as well as the body's ability to excrete them. See Appendix for protocols for testing and treatment.

LEAD

Facts

- high levels of lead in children may result in reduced hearing, muscle co-ordination and intellectual development
- lead contamination may also contribute either to lethargy or aggressive behaviour
- widely distributed throughout our environment

Contacts

- industrial sources
- past exposure to leaded gasoline (now banned)
- disposal of lead wastes
- peeling or flaking of lead-based paint
- eating fruits or vegetables grown in lead-contaminated soils
- Ontario residents are exposed every day to varying amounts of lead, through contact with contaminated soil, house dust contaminated with lead-based paint, or through local industry

Helpful tips on how to reduce your exposure to lead:

- Keep your children away from soil contaminated with lead. Contaminated soil can be removed, or exposure can be reduced by covering the soil with clean soil or sod.
- Wash children's hands and faces after they have been playing outdoors and before eating,
- Clean your home regularly using a damp mop or cloth and have forced air ducts cleaned by a professional. Of course, keep your furnace filters regularly cleaned.

CHEMICALS

- Avoid bringing outdoor dirt inside by removing outdoor shoes.
- Don't let your children eat paint chips (they like them because the lead makes them taste sweet).
- Locate your vegetable garden at least one metre away from roads, driveways and downspouts. Also make sure your garden is at least a metre away from sources of flaking paint, such as walls, sheds and fences.
- Before eating, wash all vegetables thoroughly and peel root crops.

HUMAN EXPOSURE TO LEAD

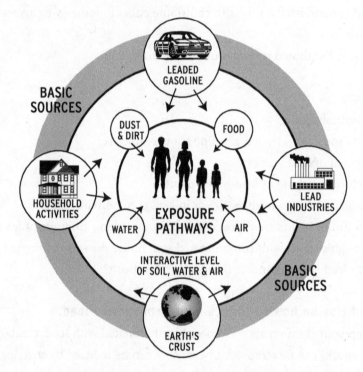

Source: Schematic representation adapted from: The Citizen's Guide to Lead: Uncovering A Hidden Health Hazard, *by Barbara Wallace and Kathy Cooper, NC Press Limited, 1986.*

ALUMINUM

Facts
- Toxic metal—believed to be implicated in Alzheimer's disease

Contacts
- Cookware, tinfoil, tin cans, drink containers. When combined with food during cooking, additional chemicals are formed;
- Acid rain soil can cause leaching of aluminum into the surrounding area;
- Waxed cardboard beverage containers may have an aluminum coating;
- In processed foods as an anticaking agent (e.g., self-rising flour, baking powder, cake mixes, processed cheese, pickles, non-dairy creams, salt, powdered foods;
- Some antacids, antidiarrheals, vaginal douches, hemorrhoidal medications, antiperspirants, lipsticks;
- Soft water, tap water.

CADMIUM

Facts
- highly toxic

Contacts
- Plating on household hardware and metal containers not intended for food, silver polish, ceramics;
- Paint pigments, polyvinyl plaster, rubber carpet backing;
- Naturally occurring in rock, cadmium can leach into water and soil;
- Tobacco smoke, cigarettes, imported lipstick, cola drinks, processed meat, freshwater fish, all seafood, bonemeal, water;
- Air pollution, incinerators, burning motor oil, smelter plants, fertilizer, fungicides, welding, cadmium batteries;

CHEMICALS

MERCURY

COMMON SOURCES

Fish and seafood, incinerators; acid rain; medications such as cathartic, diuretic, antisyphilitic, antiseptic, antipruritic, antinflammatory, antiparasitic; preservatives in eye drops, ointments, contact lens solutions, nasal sprays, vaccines, globulines.

Dental Mercury Amalgams: Annual use of mercury in the US is approximately 70,000 kg. Over 100 million mercury fillings are placed in the mouths of North Americans annually.

Damaging mercury vapour enters the brain directly, crossing the blood-brain barrier.

MERCURY EXPOSURES–WHO IS AT RISK

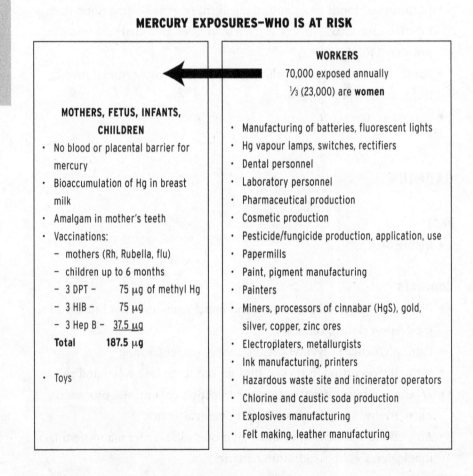

MOTHERS, FETUS, INFANTS, CHIILDREN

- No blood or placental barrier for mercury
- Bioaccumulation of Hg in breast milk
- Amalgam in mother's teeth
- Vaccinations:
  - mothers (Rh, Rubella, flu)
  - children up to 6 months
  - 3 DPT –   75 μg of methyl Hg
  - 3 HIB –   75 μg
  - 3 Hep B –   37.5 μg
  Total   187.5 μg

- Toys

WORKERS
70,000 exposed annually
⅓ (23,000) are **women**

- Manufacturing of batteries, fluorescent lights
- Hg vapour lamps, switches, rectifiers
- Dental personnel
- Laboratory personnel
- Pharmaceutical production
- Cosmetic production
- Pesticide/fungicide production, application, use
- Papermills
- Paint, pigment manufacturing
- Painters
- Miners, processors of cinnabar (HgS), gold, silver, copper, zinc ores
- Electroplaters, metallurgists
- Ink manufacturing, printers
- Hazardous waste site and incinerator operators
- Chlorine and caustic soda production
- Explosives manufacturing
- Felt making, leather manufacturing

CHEMICALS

Facts

• Highly toxic

To learn more about mercury and how it affects us, see the article on Dental Amalgams in the Special Interest section on page 296.

OXIDES

SULPHUR DIOXIDE (SO$_2$)

Facts

• Smells like burnt matches
• Results from burning of sulphur-bearing fuels
• A major contributor to acid rain
• Levels of 0.2ppm are irritating to most people

Major Sources

• Poorly vented stoves, furnaces, water heaters, and the burning of fuel oils with high sulphur contents
• Industries burning high-sulphur coal and oil
• Pulp mills
• Petrochemical refineries, smelters, diesel engines

CARBON MONOXIDE (CO)

Facts

• colourless, odourless, tasteless gas; replaces oxygen in red blood cells;
• results from incomplete combustion (gas, kerosene, wood heat, appliances, auto exhaust);

CHEMICALS

- long-term exposure at 5ppm can lead to trouble (a gas stove in a closed kitchen can exceed levels of 100ppm., a running car in a closed garage can reach levels of 1000ppm).

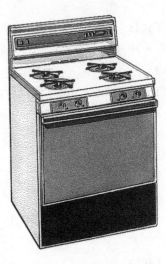

Major Sources
- Unvented, or improperly vented, combustion appliances
- Auto exhaust drawn into the house
- Tobacco smoke, candle flames, open fireplaces

Carbon Monoxide Toxicity, edited by David G. Penney, Ph.D, CRC Press Boca Raton, FL. 2000. **www.coheadquarters.com** C.O.S. Carbon Monoxide Support, 25 Swarcliffe Rd., Leeds LS14 5LE, U.K. Fax: (0113) 2281505 **www.homesafe.com/cosupport**

NITROGEN OXIDES (NO, NO$_2$)

Facts
- part of the haze in smog
- strong smell
- produced as a by-product of combustion and through the action of sunlight on polluted air
- contributes to acid rain

Major Sources
- Fuel-burning stoves, furnaces, water heaters
- Tobacco smoke, auto exhaust, industrial emissions

CHEMICALS

CARBON DIOXIDE (CO_2)

Facts
- High levels will make room feel stuffy and stale
- 2000 ppm. causes discomfort for most individuals
- 5000 ppm. leads to serious loss of alertness

Major Sources
- respiration
- combustion
- faulty chimneys and inadequate air supply to fuel-burning appliances

INDOOR POLLUTION

Health Effects and Indoor Air Quality
Almost everyone is aware of outdoor air pollution and its effect on our health. What many of us don't realize is that the air we breathe inside our homes may actually be more hazardous to our health than outside air. Modern building techniques with the increased use of synthetic, chemical-based products have resulted in increased risks to human health. The majority of our time is spent indoors, as is displayed on the chart on the next page; hence the need for improved indoor air quality.

Airborne contaminants in homes are not limited to the chemical kind; biological contaminants can originate from within the home also. Molds, another major source of trouble, grow wherever it is damp. Therefore, they can be found outside the house, in the structure of the house, and throughout the house, in obvious places like the kitchen and bathroom, and not-so-obvious places like carpets and walls.

Molds can cause chronic illnesses in humans, as well as allergic reactions and acute infections.* Formaldehyde, toluene and other volatile organic compounds (VOCs) are known to have adverse effects on human health.

* *Significance of Fungi in Indoor Air: Report of a Working Group,* Health and Welfare Canada 1987.

Below is a list of housing-related health effects as provided by *The Clean Air Guide: How to Identify and Correct Indoor Air Problems in Your Home*, a publication of the Canada Mortgage and Housing Commission, revised 1998:

Housing-Related Health Effects

Allergic rhinitis	Impaired lung function
Anemia	Impaired vision
Asthma	Impaired coordination
Asbestosis	Influenza
Cancer	Learning impairment
Cardiovascular stress	Liver and kidney damage
Coughing, sinus congestion	Loss of bone calcium
Digestive problems	Nervous system depression
Dizziness	Nose bleeds
Dry, chapped or irritated skin	Pneumonia
Emphysema	Rashes
Eye, nose, throat irritation	Respiratory distress
Fatigue	Respiratory infection
Headaches	Shortness of breath

Establishing a healthy living space is extremely important, especially as indicated by the amount of time spent indoors. It is imperative to make our homes safe, as our workplace or schools, etc., are often beyond our control.

CHEMICALS

AVERAGE DAILY TIME SPENT IN: 24-HR

Adapted from J. Robinson & G. Gody, Pennsylvania State University Press, 1997

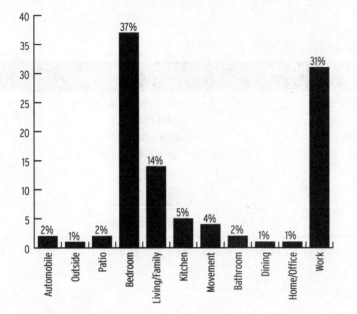

CHEMICALS

Types and Sources of Indoor Air Pollution

RESPIRABLE PARTICLES	NITROGEN DIOXIDE
• fireplaces	• gas ranges
• space heaters	• pilot lights
• coal stoves	• space heaters
• wood stoves	• gasoline engines
• tobacco smoke	• outside air
• outside air	• hockey rinks
• attached facilities	
• occupant activities	

VOCs	SEMIVOLATILE ORGANIC COMPOUNDS
• plasticizers	• pesticides
• oils	• transformer fluid
• solvents	• termiticides
• mothballs	• wood combustion
• cleaning fluids	• tobacco smoke
• glues	• kerosene

CHEMICALS

VOCs (cont.)	SEMIVOLATILE ORGANIC COMPOUNDS
• photocopiers • personal care products • resins • gasoline • formaldehyde	• wood preservative

INFECTIOUS AND ALLERGIC AGENTS	CARBON MONOXIDE
• dust mites • cockroaches • bacteria • fungi • viruses • pollen	• gas ranges • pilot lights • space heaters • gasoline engines • outside air • hockey rinks • tobacco smoke • attached garages

Adapted from "The Air Children Breathe: The Effects on Their Health" by Pollution Probe pg. 35

AVERAGE HOME COULD BE POLLUTED FROM MANY SOURCES:

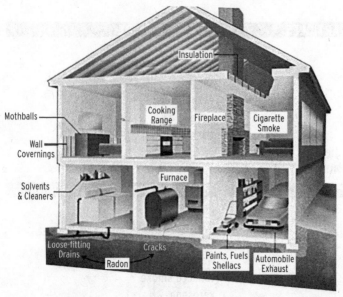

Source: Environmental Health Center —Dallas.

AIR QUALITY IN SCHOOLS

Indoor air pollution affects everyone; teachers, students, the allergic and hypersensitive individual in particular (see page 202).

Location of the School
- close to highways
- in industrial complexes
- high tension wires (effect of electromagnetic fields)
- idling school buses in front of school
- portables placed in open fields, subject to more dust and pollen

Maintenance of building
- painting and renovation during the academic year is a big contributor to indoor air pollution
- indoor pesticides
- outdoor herbicides and pesticides in the schoolyard
- unsafe chlorinated, phenolated cleaning supplies, as well as solvents and ammonia
- floor polishing, waxing
- ashphalt paving and roofing during academic year
- faulty heating and ventilation system
- scented products and air fresheners in washrooms

Classrooms
- synthetic carpets (particularly fresh, new and glued to the floor)
- furniture outgassing formaldehyde
- correction fluids
- markers containing solvents or fragrances
- paints
- chalk dust
- copy paper, carbon paper
- plastic or fiberglass drapes
- strong smelling plants

CHEMICALS

- particle board shelving
- computer terminals
- fluorescent lighting
- use of perfumes by teachers and students
- odour of tobacco from teachers and students

Vocational Courses
- poorly ventilated working areas
- large offenders for indoor air pollution in schools

Wood Working
- wood odours, sawdust
- paints, thinners, solvents, lacquers, shellac
- formaldehyde (particle board)

Mechanical Workshop
- solvents
- caulking compounds
- cleaning compounds

Industrial Arts
- heated plastics

Printing
- inks
- computers
- laminating

Home Economics
- food odours
- natural gas
- cleaning fluids

CHEMICALS

Darkroom Photography
- chemical developers

Art, Chemistry and Biology Classes
- magic markers containing solvents
- rubber or spray cement
- glue, paste
- paper products
- glaze
- paint thinners
- solvents
- oil paints
- formaldehyde
- natural gas
- Bunsen burners
- organic chemicals
- mold growth in paint cans
- poorly vented chemistry labs
- inadequate fume vent hoods in science labs

CHEMICALS

PROBLEMS CONTRIBUTING TO SICK BUILDING SYNDROME

Homes, schools, offices, and institutions which are responsible for illness of their occupants are called Sick Buildings. Symptoms caused by Sick Buildings are called Sick Building Syndrome. This was first officially defined by the World Health Organization (WHO) in 1983.

- inadequate or complete lack of maintenance of existing ventilation systems due to lack of funds, etc. (effective maintenance is expensive)
- introduction to the building of new equipment or activities for which original ventilation systems were not designed
- changing policies on standards of ventilation in the building
- 70–80% of contaminated air merely recycled (only 20% fresh air added to ventilation)

- some architectural designs and ventilation designs are faulty in themselves:
    - open concept of offices: use of partitions
    - "well" type of construction
    - intake of air close to exhausts
    - intake of air from parking lots
    - use of contaminated water for humidification of air
- contamination of air from inadequately vented underground parking
- switching off ventilation systems on the weekend
- lack of ventilation and/or cross contamination of air from tobacco designated areas
- indoor use of pest control
    - every 6 weeks to every 6 months, depending on level of activity
    - banks, nursing homes use pest control every 6 weeks
    - some restaurant kitchens and cafeterias use it weekly
- broadloom (the most unhygienic invention of the last century)
    - major collectors of dust, dirt, bacteria, viruses and toxic chemicals; particularly dangerous if new and glued down
    - use of carpet fresheners
    - no cleaning method is adequate
- cleaning services
    - use of chlorinated, phenol containing compounds and solvents
- plants*
    - mold often grows on the soil surface
    - maintenance may require use of fungicides and pesticides
    - use of shiners contaminates the air

*some plants can be used as formaldehyde and/or other toxin absorbers, provided that the soil is covered with activated charcoal to prevent mold contamination from the soil (see page 190)

- renovation in offices with inadequate protection of individuals in the same space or adjacent offices
    - formaldehydes, paints, solvents, caulking materials, glues, new carpets, etc., are all hazardous to health from 2 weeks to 8 months

CHEMICALS

after renovation, depending on the type of material used and
ventilation systems in place

- partitions made of synthetic fabrics—same problem as carpets
- different hazardous activities in buildings with inadequate (or lack of)
existing exhausting and ventilation systems
  - photography (formaldehyde)
  - copying facilities (solvents)
  - dry cleaning (solvents)
  - laminations (heated plastic, phtalates)
- computers
  - electromagnetic radiation from video terminals, wires,
    transmitters, etc.
  - some people are surrounded by them from all sides
  - outgassing from heated plastic parts
- office supplies
  - newsprint, papers, carbonless paper, liquid paper, markers, rubber
    bands, copying machine toners and solvents, etc.
- personal use scented products
  - perfumes, colognes, hair sprays, shampoo, conditioners,
    deodorizers, detergents, fabric softeners

**The majority of these products used at home, office and school, not only
affect health but also decrease productivity.** The chemicals mentioned
belong to the three previously mentioned categories of pollutants, such as
formaldehyde, synthetic ethyl alcohol and phenols.

TOBACCO SMOKE

Tobacco smoke is a definite health hazard both to the smoker and the non-
smoker. In addition to the known relationship between tobacco smoke and
lung cancer, consider that tobacco smoke contains over 1,200 chemicals,
60 of which are known carcinogens. The dried leaf is treated with many

CHEMICALS

chemicals to pass on aroma and flavour; sugar is added for taste. In addition, the plant is sprayed with poisonous insecticides, and the cigarette is composed of chemically treated paper; the burning of which releases even more contaminants. Note that both inhaled smoke and cigarettes left burning are a problem. In short, tobacco smoking interferes with any possibility of improvement, especially for the hypersensitive, whether they or someone they live with smokes.

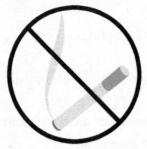

IF YOU SMOKE, DON'T EXHALE!

Tobacco Smoke and Children:

It was known by 1986 that children of smokers have a 20% to 80% greater risk of developing respiratory problems, such as asthma, bronchitis, and pneumonia, than do children of non-smokers. Some researchers now speculate that smoke from a father's cigarette inhaled by a smoking or non-smoking mother may have the same effect on the fetus as maternal smoking.

By the 1970s it was known that eight million people with common allergies are also clinically sensitive to tobacco.

PERFUMES/FRAGRANCES

The ingredients in perfumes are dangerous chemicals, no less so than those found in tobacco smoke. Fragrances are made up of volatile organic compounds, which can affect not only the respiratory system, but the central nervous system as well. "Scents" are now widely used, and the number of products being perfumed is increasing, while there has been little research into the effects of inhaling fragrances. Most testing is for dermatological reactions of primary users. There is little data on carcinogenic or neurotoxic effects or potential effects on fetal development.

Perfumes often present a major obstacle for people with asthma, allergies, sensitivities, and chronic severe headaches. Fragrance topped the list of frustrations faced by people with exposure-related health problems, according to a 1997 HEAL (Human Ecology Action League) member survey. Although many scent-free policies are being put into place voluntarily, not enough workplaces are cooperative to the needs of sensitive individuals. Such places of employment as hospitals, nursing homes, medical clinics, daycare

CHEMICALS

irritability
mental vagueness
asthma bloating joint aches muscle pain
sinus pain
sore throat   fatigue
eye irritation
         gastrointestinal problems
laryngitis   headaches   dizziness
swollen lymph nodes   lost thoughts
spiked blood pressure   coughing
burning, itching skin eruptions

ETHANOL   BENZALDEHYDE
BENZYL ACETATE   a-PINENE
CAMPHOR   ACETONE
BENZYL ALCOHOL   ETHYL ACETATE
LINALOOL   LIMONENE
METHYLENE CHLORIDE
a-TERPINENE
a-TERPINEOL

**THE MOST COMMON CHEMICALS FOUND
IN FRAGRANCE PRODUCTS AND
SOME OF THEIR EFFECTS**

Source: Health hazards information compiled by Julia Kendall. Full info available on www.ehnca.org. Adapted from B. Wilkie.

facilities, schools, government services, places of worship, food handlers and restaurants, should all advocate a "no scent" policy. I trust that one day perfumes will follow the fate of tobacco.

Some regard perfume as simply a pleasant fragrance, not realizing that they are also applying and inhaling a number of synthetic compounds. There are sometimes between ten and one hundred compounds that are volatile or airborne in perfumes. Chemicals include acetone, ethanol, limonene, toluene, phenol, benzaldehyde, benzylacetate, benzyl alcohol, camphor, ethyl acetate, methyl chloride, pinene, terpinene, toluene, linlool, etc., with resultant health effects including dizziness, nausea, slurred speech, respiratory and eye irritation.

Although it is widely accepted that allergic reactions, especially asthma, can be aggravated by perfumes acting as an irritant to the inflamed airways of the allergic sufferer; environmental illnesses, such as chronic fatigue syndrome, multiple chemical sensitivity and fibromyalgia, do not get the consideration they deserve in the matter of fragrances.

Resources: Environmental Health Network: www.ehnca.org. Fragranced Products Information Network: www.fpinva.org

Environmental Correction (see also p. 205)

- **Home** – Perfumes need not be used at all (including personal care products)—seek out and use products with no fragrance, or very low residual fragrance.
  – Do not use air fresheners or other environmental fragrance products in the home.
  – Do not use scented cleaning products or fabric conditioners.
- **School** – Staff should be encouraged not to wear perfume.
  – Introduce "no scent" policy.
  – Encourage scent-free cleaning products.
- **Office** – Office personnel should be encouraged not to wear perfume. Having an allergic reaction or an asthmatic attack in the office because of others' perfume is not a pleasant or necessary experience.

PLASTICS

These man-made substances constantly outgas, particularly when heated. The general rule of thumb is the more flexible and odourous a new plastic, the more likely it is to cause problems. With this in mind, the worst offenders are soft plastics, such as shower curtains, tablecloths, toys, shopping bags, upholstery materials, combs, brushes, pillow and mattress cases, handbags, shoes, plastic wrap, and so on. See also Hormone Disrupting Chemicals (page 270) and also Cancer Causes and Prevention (page 301).

Forms of Plastic

- Acrylonitrile (Lucite/Plexiglass)
- Epoxy Resins
- Latex (see next page)
- Nylon
- Phenol-Formaldehyde (Bakelite)
- Polyester—this material releases the most fumes
- Polyurethane—releases toluene disocyanate that can cause pulmonary, skin and eye problems
- Polyvinyl chloride (PVC)—releases vinyl chloride
- Polyvinylpyrrolidone (PVP)—in hairspray
- Tetrafluoroethylene (Teflon)—produces poisonous gases when burnt, possibly when heated
- Polystyrene (styrofoam)

Plasticizers

- chemicals (phthalates, Bisphenol A) added to plastic to keep it soft and flexible (the new car smell, toys, etc.).

Contacts

- Plastic food storage containers and plastic wrap contaminate food through the migration of plasticizers. This occurs even more readily when the containers are heated or used in a microwave.

CHEMICALS

- Contact lenses/eye glasses, hair and tooth brushes
- Lamp shades, often coated in plastic, which is particularly offensive when heated by the bulb.
- Rug pads, bakelite handles on pots, self-stick shelf paper (may also have added pesticides), shower curtains, plastic coated papers, teflon, SilveStone plastic coatings on pots, irons, ironing board covers, plastic wrap for clothing, furniture, toys, food, etc.

Latex Allergy

Latex allergy has recently become a major problem for many individuals, particularly health care workers, as they are exposed to natural rubber latex from gloves used in medical and dental practices. Latex is made from the sap of the rubber tree (Hevea brasiliensis). Latex allergy often begins with a rash on the hands when using natural rubber latex gloves. Other allergic symptoms include hay fever type reactions, such as itchy swollen eyes, runny nose, and sneezing. Some individuals may develop asthma symptoms, such as chest tightness, wheezing, coughing, shortness of breath, and although uncommon, even anaphylactic reactions.

Probably the best advice for someone with a latex allergy is "avoidance." Avoid contact with natural rubber latex products such as those listed in the table on the next page. Non-latex substitutes are available for most commonly used natural rubber latex products. Remember to contact your doctor or dentist before your visit to warn them of your latex allergy. If you work in high latex exposure areas and have skin irritation, hay fever or asthma symptoms, you should advise your employer and consult a physician about your treatment. Obtain and wear a Medic Alert bracelet if your allergy is severe. Prior to surgery, you should consult your physician about the need for a latex-free operating environment.

CHEMICALS

NATURAL RUBBER LATEX PRODUCTS	SUBSTITUTES
For Babies–pacifiers, feeding nipples	Silicone products
For School and Office–erasers, craft supplies, make-up and Halloween masks, adhesives	Look for products labelled "vinyl" or "silicone"
Clothing–elastic fabric, diapers, underwear	Many elastic fabrics are not rubber (for instance "Spandex" and "Lycra"), but elastic webbing often contains rubber
Housework–cleaning gloves	Gloves are a major source of exposure because they are in direct contact with the skin for a long time and may give off an allergenic dust–use nitrile, neoprene, vinyl or copolymer gloves
Toys and Sporting Goods–balloons, rubber ducks, soccer balls, volleyballs, coated or taped racquet handles	Mylar (foil type) balloons, leather balls
Furnishings–rubber mats, carpet backing, foam rubber	Most foam rubber is polyurethane foam and will not cause problems
Medical Products	
- condoms, female condoms, diaphragms	Synthetic rubber or natural membrane condoms
- medical gloves, dental dams	As with household gloves above, use only gloves made with synthetic materials
- first aid tape, bandages	Some brands do not contain natural rubber latex
- surgical products , blood pressure cuffs, catheters, etc.	Your doctor will have access to non-latex substitutes

CHEMICALS

(Medical Devices Bureau, Health Protection Branch, Health Canada 1-800-267-9675. This chart was adapted from a Guideline for Allergic Patients produced by the Canadian Society of Allergy and Clinical Immunology (CSACI) called Natural Rubber Latex Allergy.

CHEMICALS

FABRICS

Generally speaking, natural fibres are more satisfactory for clothing, linens and furnishings than materials that have to be artificially processed. Synthetic fabrics are bothersome not only because they are derived from petroleum, but also because they hold electrical charges (static) and will attract unwanted pollution particles. It is important to use untreated natural fibres as any of the following treatments involve the use of formaldehyde, plastic resins, and so on: water repellent, stain resistant, flame resistant, wrinkle resistant, moth proof, crush proof, increased elasticity, and permanent press.

Other factors to consider when choosing a fabric are:
- bonded fabrics involve the use of glue
- imported fabrics are often sprayed with pesticides
- bleaching alters the fabric and may be bothersome
- many cottons are sized with polyester resin
- dyes are set in conjunction with formaldehyde, the more intense the colour the more troublesome
- fabrics for ironing boards can be teflon coated

Synthetic Fibres (Petroleum Based)
- Nylon, rayon, acetate, acrilon, acrylic, orlon, dacron, polyester
- Nylon is the least offensive and polyester the most
- Some rayons, rayon/viscose are produced from wood fibres, possibly containing pine tree resins

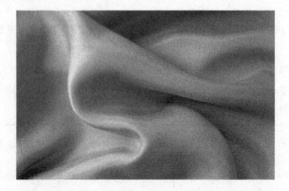

Natural Fibres

- Cotton, linen, wool, silk, and blends of these

Below is a table that describes the classification of fibres

CLASSIFICATION OF FIBRES

NATURAL FIBRES	MAN-MADE FIBRES
Vegetable	Well tolerated
· Seed–cotton, kapok	· Inorganic–glass, rock, slag,
· Bast–flax/linen, ramie, jute, hemp, Indian mallow, kenaf	tinsel thread
· Leaf–abaca, sisal, Zealand hemp, cantala	
· Fruit–coir	
Mineral	Reasonably well tolerated
· Asbestos–dangerous, carcinogenic, never to be used	· Regenerated–cellulose base e.g., viscose rayon, protein base
	· Semi-synthetic–cellulose base e.g., acetate, acetylated rayon
Animal	Poorly tolerated
· Silk-insects	· Synthetic–polymerization
· Hair-wool, goat (mohair, cashmere, goat hair), camel (camel, vicuna, alpaca), llama, horse	e.g., polyethylene, polyvinyl, polyacrylonitrile (Acrylic)

CHEMICALS

CLOTHING

- Nickel or other metals in undergarments can be troublesome.
- Nylon garments are often plastic coated.
- Dry-cleaning processes leave residues.
- Rubber in bras and elastic topped underwear can cause problems.
- Bleaches, fabric softeners, antistatic agents used in home laundry products can never be completely washed out.

- Clothing picks up odours very easily. (For this reason, keep soiled clothing out of the room in which you sleep.)
- Old synthetics may be tolerable due to repeated washings.
- Vinyl and leather articles of clothing can emit strong odours.

IMPORTANT NOTE:

AS DISCUSSED IN THE INTRODUCTION, ALL CHEMICALS ENTER THE BODY THROUGH VARIOUS ROUTES OF EXPOSURE AND ARE THEN METABOLIZED BY THE BODY. WHEN THE DETOXIFYING ENZYME SYSTEM IS WEAK, PROBLEM CHEMICALS ARE DEPOSITED IN FAT TISSUE. THEY ARE THEN SLOWLY RELEASED FROM THE FAT TISSUE INTO THE BLOODSTREAM, THUS POISONING THE HUMAN SYSTEM AND FORMING THE BASIS FOR MANY OF THE DEGENERATIVE DISEASES IN MODERN SOCIETY.

CHEMICALS

Food and Nutrition

FOOD FOR THOUGHT

Many environmentally sensitive individuals discover that they react to food they eat. It might be the food itself, a chemical used at some stage of its production, or one of the naturally occurring chemicals found within foods (see natural phenols, page 104). The following pages will touch upon the concept of food sensitivities and the quality of foods we ingest. More specifically, we will look at common contacts with, and alternatives to, allergenic foods.

FOOD ALLERGY	FOOD SENSITIVITY, FOOD INTOLERANCE
• Immunologically mediated reactions (mainly IgE)	• Non-IgE immunologically mediated reactions (IgG immune complexes, etc.)
• These food allergens often produce anaphylaxis (e.g., peanut, fish, seafood and nuts)	• Non-immunological reactions due to:
	- toxic substance (e.g., caffeine)
	- enzyme defect (e.g., lactase)
	- aspect of the food (e.g., acidic)
	- plus other possibilities (e.g., chemical contamination

Food allergy and food sensitivity both result in a definite cause-and-effect relationship between a food and the production of symptoms. Non-immunological responses appear to be more prevalent; but, in some cases, additional stress is being placed on the individual's body. Avoidance is the key to reducing that stress.

Note: In the following pages, the term *food sensitivity* will be used to indicate a problem with a food without differentiating as to the cause of the reaction.

TOTAL BODY LOAD AND FOOD REACTIONS

The more stressors, the more difficult for your body to function effectively, and the greater the possibility of a reaction.

Some factors that can influence food sensitivity:

- speed of ingestion, which is accelerated by alcoholic beverages
- degree of usage
- food combinations
- cold, light, heat
- fatigue can accentuate symptoms
- potential of food for sensitization
- other seasonal sensitivities—cross-reaction of food with pollens
- condition of food—raw or cooked

Note: Some sensitive individuals can be bothered and become sick just by the smell of food alone.

Any food can cause reactions; however, the following foods are particularly common food allergens:

- cow's milk
- cane sugar
- orange
- nuts (particularly coconut)
- wheat
- shellfish
- soybeans
- chocolate

- corn
- peanuts
- pork
- beef

- eggs
- fish
- berries

As hard as it is to believe, the more you like a particular food, the more often you eat it or crave it, the more likely it is to be the problem food causing reactions.

CYCLICAL FOOD SENSITIVITIES

Fortunately, the majority of food sensitivities are cyclical. In such cases, after a period of strict avoidance, (usually three months for children and six months for adults), the offending food can be reintroduced on a rotational basis. However, over-indulgence may lead to the food's once again causing reactions. The difficulty lies in the fact that the reaction may not be the same as before, presenting with different symptoms. This may lead the patient to think that something else is causing the reaction or illness. It's best to go back and review the food-eating pattern and preferably reintroduce the rotation diet (see page 222).

FIXED FOOD SENSITIVITIES

In contrast, fixed food sensitivities will not change; no matter how long a food has been avoided, or how little is eaten.

ANAPHYLAXIS

Anaphylaxis is a severe, life-threatening reaction characterized by a drop in blood pressure that, if not treated immediately, can result in death. Foods to which you are anaphylactic must be avoided for life, and it is recommended that you carry an Epi-Pen with you at all times.

FOOD AND NUTRITION

DO YOU CRAVE CERTAIN FOODS?

Well, you are not alone. In fact, many people experience cravings for foods to which they have hidden sensitivities. In the process of trying to adapt to the problem food, the body may become addicted. If this is the case, an individual may actually feel worse if they don't receive their daily supply of the offending food. A great deal of stress is placed on the body as it tries to cope with these foods. So, even though one may temporarily feel better, the long-term effect is not positive. The good news is that after a period of avoidance (usually two weeks), physical cravings and withdrawal symptoms subside. It takes at least three months for children and six months for adults to regain tolerance of an offending food, so that it may be reintroduced on a rotational basis without producing symptoms.

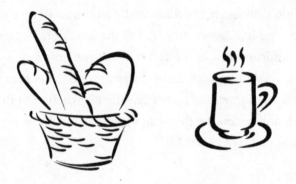

The following pyramid simply indicates that foods can be addictive. They contain phenolic compounds, some of which are opiates. Some drugs contain food incipients (lactose, glucose, corn) which are addictive. Drugs, natural or synthetic (morphine, heroin), or related chemical exposures, all contribute to addictions of all sorts and can lead to obesity. The smaller the molecular weight, the heavier the addiction. Recently, the discovery that the hormone Peptide YY3-36, made by cells in the small intestine in response to food and carried to our brain, can switch off the craving urge for food has shed additional light on this phenomenon.

Ref: Stephen Bloom, et al. Nature 418, Vol. 6898, pages 650–654, 2002. The gut hormone PYY3-36 physiologically inhibits food intake.

THE ADDICTION PYRAMID

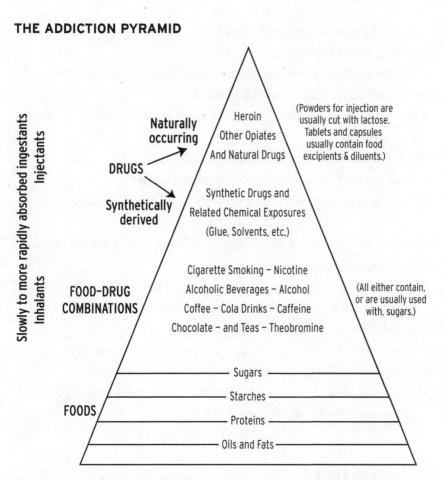

The Addiction Pyramid: Source: Randolph, Theron. Environmental Medicine—Beginnings and Bibliographies of Clinical Ecology, *Fort Collins, CO: Clinical Ecology Publications, Inc.* 1987. pg. 251.

DIGESTION OF A FOOD

The body requires oxygen, carbohydrates, fats, protein, minerals, vitamins and water in order to function. We derive these nutrients from the air we breathe and from every-day food and drink; then digestive processes break them down into forms accessible to our body cells. Keep in mind that a reaction can occur at any point during the digestion of food. A study conducted on 376 patients found that the earliest reaction occurred in three minutes.

All individuals reported symptoms within one hour, and 72% had a reaction within thirty minutes.

The length of time required for the digestive process varies according to age, the individual, and the nature of the food.

- From mouth to stomach, solids take seven seconds and liquids take four seconds
- Time in stomach—approximately three hours
- Time in small intestine—approximately six hours
- Time in large intestine—approximately ten to thirteen hours

Other important processes beside digestion play a role in the maintenance of proper nutrition:

- absorption, through mucous membranes, of digested foods, which are then transported by blood and lymph to all organs
- assimilation of nutrients by different organs
- elimination through the G.I. tract, kidney, lungs and skin (a proper bowel movement is essential for the well-being of the person)
- Any of the above mentioned is dependent upon the energetic processes of the entire body's metabolism.

CARBOHYDRATES

Roles of Carbohydrates

- provide the body with energy (brain cannot use any other source of energy)
- protein-sparing because the body does not have to burn protein for energy when carbohydrates are present
- assist in the breakdown of body fat to energy
- energy provided is used to build, maintain and repair; also to heat the body and supply muscles with needed energy

Facts

- Carbohydrates = carbon, hydrogen, oxygen
- the number and arrangement of the components dictates the type of carbohydrate.

Simple Carbohydrates:

- monosaccharides   glucose, fructose, galactose
- disaccharides   sucrose (glucose + fructose)
- lactose (glucose + galactose)
- maltose (glucose + glucose)

Complex Carbohydrates:

- starches (energy storage in plants)
- glycogen (energy storage in animals)
- fibre (structural part of plant)
- during digestion, all carbohydrates are broken down into glucose; the blood then transports this to body cells, where the energy can be utilized
- excess carbohydrates are stored as glycogen for short-term needs and as fat deposits for long-term requirements

Recommended Nutrient Intake for Canadians

- carbohydrates, with an emphasis on the complex variety, should comprise 60% of daily caloric intake
- a maximum of 10 grams of simple carbohydrates per day
- between 15-30 grams of fibre per day

Foods High in Simple Sugars

- refined sugars
- concentrated sweeteners, e.g., maple syrup, honey
- fruit juice, milk, vegetables

FOOD AND NUTRITION

Foods High in Complex Carbohydrates
- roots and tubers
- unrefined whole grains
- legumes
- nuts and seeds

PROTEINS

Roles of Proteins
- provide the basic building blocks (amino acids) for the structural material of the body (building and rebuilding of body cells)
- can be burnt as fuel if no carbohydrates are present, but this occurs at a price to the body
- produce enzymes that assist with essential body functions e.g., digestion, detoxification, etc.

Facts
- protein = chain of amino acids
- there are eight amino acids considered "essential" as they can only be provided by food: valine, leucine, isoleucine, lysine, methionine, treomine, phenylalanine, tryptophan
- protein-rich foods also contain fats and carbohydrates (no one nutrient stands alone in any food source)
- protein from plants is incomplete
- **complementary proteins** involve two or more vegetable sources of protein which, when eaten individually, are lacking in an essential amino acid but, when eaten together, supply a full complement.
- Complementary protein combinations include:
  - legumes + grains (e.g., kidney beans on rice)
  - legumes + nuts or seeds (e.g., chick pea patties + tahini)
  - grains + nuts or seeds (e.g., almond butter on rye crackers)

- dairy + grains (e.g., oatmeal with goat's milk)
- dairy + nuts or seeds (e.g., yogurt with walnuts or flaxseed)
- Proper intake of complementary proteins is essential in vegetarian diets

Recommended Nutrient Intake for Canadians
- Proteins should comprise at least 10 % of daily caloric intake

LIPIDS

Roles of Fats
- efficient storage of energy (carbohydrates must be present to burn it effectively)
- supply essential fats and fat-soluble vitamins
- add taste and aroma to foods
- protect body organs and provides insulating layer
- provide feeling of fullness

Facts
- Lipid = 1 glycerol molecule + fatty acid molecules
- Number and configuration of the fatty acids provide the characteristics of the lipid
- Triglycerides are the most common; they are made up of 3 fatty acids
- Diglycerides = 2 fatty acids, monoglycerides = 1 fatty acid
- Phospholipids are found in food and in our body. They are made up of 1 glycerol + 2 fatty acids + 1 phosphorus-containing acid, they play a role in the health of cell membranes, lethicin is a phospholipid
- Cholesterol is manufactured in animals. It is the base for production of some hormones. It can accumulate along the blood transportation system. Blood cholesterol, not dietary cholesterol, is an indicator of potential difficulties
- Polyunsaturated fats help reduce blood cholesterol

- Dietary cholesterol intake should be no more than 300 mg per day
- **Essential fatty acids (EFAs)**: refers to those fats that the body cannot manufacture itself; linoleic acid and linolenic acid. These are found in fish and vegetable oils. EFAs play an integral role in every single cell of the body, and are especially important for the function of the brain. They are necessary for adults and particularly children.
- Cold pressed: refers to oils with minimal processing, and therefore greater retention of nutrients.

A concise and helpful guide to proper use of oils can be found in the following book: *Good Fats and Oils* by Siegfried Gursche, (Alive Books, 2000).

An excellent book on essential fatty acids is *Phospholipid Spectrum Disorder in Psychiatry* by Glen Peet and David Horrobin, (Marius, U.K. 1999).

Configuration of Lipids

SATURATED	UNSATURATED	HYDROGENATED
• All available carbon bonds are filled with hydrogen	• Not completely filled with hydrogen	• Hydrogen is added to unsaturated fats, filling the available bonds and creating saturated fat
• Generally solid at room temperature	• Monounsaturated–one hydrogen missing, e.g., olive	
• Come from animal sources and some plants e.g., coconut, palm and palm kernel oils	• Polyunsaturated–more than one hydrogen missing, e.g., safflower	• This is done to make the liquid more solid and to help preserve it
• It is recommended that only 10% of fat intake be saturated	• Generally liquid at room temperature	• An example is margarine
	• Prone to rancidity	
	• Extremely important for function of arteries, brain and every cell membrane	

Margarine, an example of a hydrogenated fat, is a source of trans fatty acids, which represent a major dietary risk factor for premature heart disease. Like saturated fats, trans fats raise LDL cholesterol ("bad" cholesterol), but they're even more harmful because they also lower the HDL or "good" cholesterol. They also may stiffen the cell membrane leading to impaired function.

The **P:S Ratio** refers to the ratio of polyunsaturated fats compared to saturated fats. The higher the ratio, the better the oil. Below are listed some oils and their P:S ratio:

Safflower	7:1
Sunflower	4:1
Corn/soy	3:1
Peanut	1:1

RECOMMENDED NUTRIENT INTAKE FOR CANADIANS

- Health Canada recommends that you get no more than 30% of your daily calories from fats
- Reduce fat intake and increase P:S ratio (fat is linked to cancer when eaten in excess; polyunsaturated fats lower blood cholesterol)
- Your body needs a certain amount of fat for energy and essential fatty acids for specific metabolic functions. Fat helps your body absorb and use important fat-soluble vitamins A, D, E, and K and some types of fatty acids, e.g., Omega-3, actually protect against heart disease. Just be wise in your choice; stay away from margarine, and stay within the 30% recommended amount.

FOOD AND NUTRITION

Fat Content of Some Common Foods

HIGH FAT CONTENT	MODERATE FAT CONTENT	LOW FAT CONTENT
• cream cheese	• beef, pork, lamb (lean meat only)	• fish, shellfish (baked, broiled, steamed)
• hot dogs		• bread, bagels, English muffins
• peanut butter	• eggs, boiled or poached	
• luncheon meats		• legumes
• eggs, fried or scrambled	• organ meats (kidney, heart, liver)	• skim milk
• ground beef	• canned salmon, tuna (oil packed)	• all fruits and juices
• chicken wings		
• spareribs		

Note: When a label indicates "vegetable oil," it can be from any number of sources, the most common being soy, peanut, coconut, corn, and palm. Lard generally comes from pork.

QUALITY LEVELS OF EATING

Remember: the least processed and stored organic food is the best source of vitamins, minerals, essential oils and antioxidants. Try to eat as much as possible from Levels 1 and 2.

> 1. As Mother Nature created it, with nothing added and minimal preparation. **Fresh.**
>
>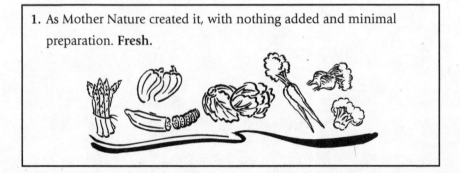

2. Lightly cooked whole foods with no preservatives.

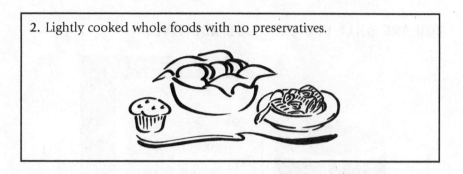

3. Cooked, canned or frozen, commercially prepared food with minimal additives.

- Fruit in own syrup
- Frozen/canned
- Pasta
- White flour
- Drug-free meats

- Powdered eggs
- Creamed cottage cheese
- Dry roasted nuts
- Frozen/canned fish

4. Highly refined, processed, packaged foods.

Source: Prof. Ross Hume Hall.

FOOD AND NUTRITION

YOU ARE WHAT YOU EAT—FOOD ADDITIVES

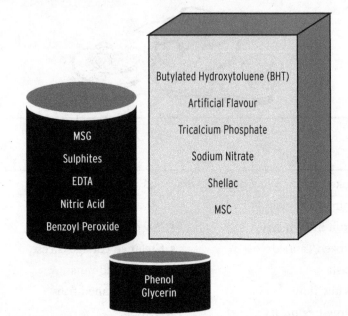

Butylated Hydroxytoluene (BHT)

Artificial Flavour

Tricalcium Phosphate

Sodium Nitrate

Shellac

MSC

MSG
Sulphites
EDTA
Nitric Acid
Benzoyl Peroxide

Phenol
Glycerin

FOOD AND NUTRITION

In an effort to produce more cosmetically pleasing, long-lasting, and convenient foods, the food and agriculture industries modify the natural state of our daily bread. In fact so do we, each time we chop, whip, cook or otherwise transform our groceries into dinner. Any amount of "processing" will have a detrimental effect upon the nutrients contained within a food, nutrients essential to the effective functioning of the human body. For this reason alone, we owe it to ourselves to seriously study the quality and contents of the foods we eat, beginning with the processing that takes place in our kitchen. The previous page outlines quality levels of food preparation, level one being the highest and four the lowest.

AN APPLE A DAY MAY NOT KEEP THE DOCTOR AWAY!

The story of the commercially produced apple pie from tree to plate.

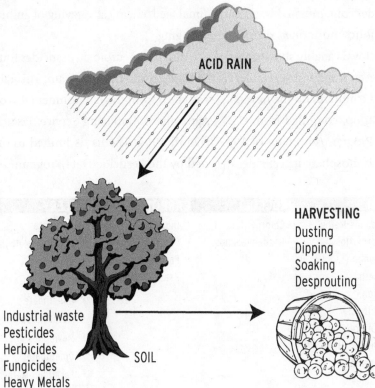

ACID RAIN

HARVESTING
Dusting
Dipping
Soaking
Desprouting

Industrial waste
Pesticides
Herbicides
Fungicides
Heavy Metals

SOIL

PROCESSING/LOSS OF NUTRIENTS

+ colouring, flavouring, flavour enhancers, bleaching, maturing, texture agents, conditioning, anti-caking, acid/base balancing additives, firming agents, enrichers

PACKAGING

gassing, waxing, colouring, Irradiation

+ possible plastic residues, preservatives

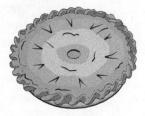

The average apple is sprayed with pesticides seventeen times, from bud stage in the spring until harvest time.

And the picture isn't much better for animal-source foods, when you consider contaminated water and animal feed, chemical spraying of animals, antibiotics, hormones, drugs and packaging.

Below is a table showing seventeen different neurotoxic pesticides found on eleven fruits and vegetables by the US Pesticide Data Program. This table, which continues on the next page, was taken from the Environmental Working Group, compiled from USDA Agricultural Marketing Service, Pesticide Data Program summary of 1992 in April 1994. The list is limited to only organophosphate insecticides detected by the Pesticide Data Program.

APPLES	BROCCOLI	CARROTS	CELERY
• Azinphos-Methyl	• Chlorpyrifos	• Diazinon	• Acephate
• Chlorpyrifos	• Methamidaphos	• Demethoate	• Azinphos-Methyl
• Diazinon		• Parathion	• Chlorpyrifos
• Dimethoate		• Paathion-Methyl	• Diazinon
• Ethion			• Dimethoate
• Omethoate			• Methamidaphos
• Parathion			• Mevinphos
• Parathion-Methyl			• Omethoate
• Phosalone			• Parathion-Methyl
• Phosmet			

GRAPEFRUIT	GRAPES	GREEN BEANS	LETTUCE
• Chlorpyrifos	• Azinphos-Methyl	• Acephate	• Acephate
• Diazinon	• Chlorpyrifos	• Azinphos-Methyl	• Chlorpyrifos
• Ethion	• Diazinon	• Chlorpyrifos	• Diazinon
• Phosmet	• Dimethoate	• Demeton	• Dimethoate
	• Methamidaphos	• Demeton-Sulfone	• Disolfoton Sulfone
	• Mevinphos	• Diazinon	• Methamidaphos
	• Omethoate	• Dimethoate	• Mevinphos
	• Parathion	• Ethion	• Omethoate
	• Parathion-Methyl	• Methamidaphos	• Parathion-Methyl
	• Phosmet	• Omethoate	
		• Parathion	
		• Parathion-Methyl	

ORANGES	PEACHES	POTATOES
• Chlorpyrifos	• Acephate	• Azinphos-Methyl
• Diazinon	• Azinphos-Methyl	• Diazinon
• Mimethoate	• Chlorpyrifos	• Demethoate
• Ethion	• Diazinon	• Methadathion
• Methadathion	• Dimethoate	• Methamidaphos
• Omethoate	• Methamidaphos	• Phorate Sulfone
	• Mevinphos	
	• Parathion	
	• Parathion-Methyl	
	• Phosmet	

It is always preferable to eat organic food.

Individuals are increasingly turning to organic foods and avoiding packaged/processed foods in favour of the homemade meal, and with good reason. (Refer to the section on Pesticides, Herbicides and Fungicides on page 93, and Hormone Disrupting Chemicals on page 270 for more information).

ORGANIC FOODS

The better the soil, the better crops and food. Without soil, we would have no air to breathe, no clean water to drink and no food to eat. Soil is indispensable and sustains us. The biology of soil is more complicated than other ecosystems as it contains most of the earth's biodiversity. One teaspoon of top soil contains more than one million bacteria, forty miles of fungi, hundreds of thousands of amoeba, hundreds of tiny worms. All work hard at shredding and decomposing so that we can live. Globally, surface soil holds twice the amount of carbon than that of all earth's vegetation and atmosphere together. Tampering with soil could have a global effect on climate as well.

Organic farming, producing organic foods, eliminates pesticides, fertilizers, antibiotics and growth hormones (except those allowed by the organic certification standards of certification agencies) and not using genetically modified plants, promotes the use of crop rotations and cover crops, and encourages balanced host/predator relationships.

Disallowed products and practices must not be employed for at least three years prior to harvest in order to be labelled certified organic. And livestock must be raised organically and fed 100% organic feeds for at least twelve months before slaughtering.

Organic foods not only contain fewer chemicals (no food is completely uncontaminated today) and taste better, they also contain more nutrients.

Mean percent additional mineral content in organic compared to conventional crops

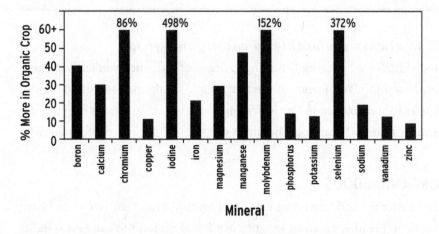

Differences in Nutritional Content Between Organic and Conventional Vegetables: Mean Percent Difference for Four Nutrients in Five Frequently Studied Vegetables

	NUTRIENT*			
VEGETABLE	VITAMIN C	IRON	MAGNESIUM	PHOSPHORUS
Lettuce	+17	+17	+29	+14
Spinach	+52	+25	-13	+14
Carrot	-6	+12	+69	+13
Potato	+22	+21	+5	0
Cabbage	+43	+41	+40	+22

*Plus and minus signs refer to conventional crops as the baseline for comparison. For example, vitamin C is 17.0% more abundant in organic lettuce (conventional 100%, organic 117%).

Source: Worthington, V. *Nutritional Quality of Organic Versus Conventional Fruits, Vegetables and Grains.* The Journal of Alternative and Complementary Medicine, Vol. 7, No. 2, 2001, pp 161–173 available at http://www.organics.comorganic_info/articles/downloads/organic/pdf

Any individual with severe chemical sensitivities should eat organic food exclusively to help in recovery.

Figure 1. Organic vs Conventional

Percent of 1230 published comparisons where nutrient levels are better, worse or the same.

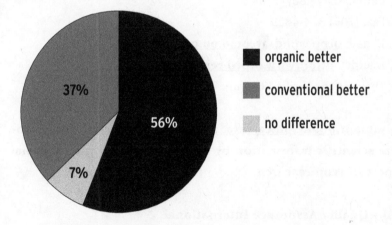

Source: V. Worthington. Nutrition and Biodynamics: Evidence for the Nutritional Superiority of Organic Crops. Biodynamics v. 224, July/August 1999.

FOOD AND NUTRITION

CERTIFICATION BODIES

OCIA—Organic Crop Improvement Association

1340 North Cotner

Lincoln, NE 68505   USA

Internet: **http://www.ocia.org**

OCIA has over 60 chapters worldwide (most in North America). They use the Certified Organic trademark.

OCPP—Organic Crop Producers and Processors Ontario Inc.

OCPP/Pro-Cert Canada UBC.

c/o Larry Lenhardt, R. R. #1, 1099 Monarch Rd., Lindsay,

Ontario K9V 4R1

Phone: (877) 867-4264

Fax: (705) 324-4829

E-mail: **ocpp@lindsaycomp.on.ca**

Internet: **http://www.ocpro-certcanada.com**

They use the Verified Organic trademark.

www.plant.uoguelph.ca/research/homepages/eclark for up-to-date scientific information by Prof. A. Clark, an international expert in crop research.

QAI—Quality Assurance International

Organic Certification

9191 Towne Center Drive, Suite 510, San Diego, CA 92122 USA

Tel: (858) 792-3531

Fax: (858) 792-8665

E-mail: **qai@qai-inc.com**

Internet: **http://www.qai-inc.com**

Canada Representative: Kasey Moctezuma

Phone: (858) 792-3531

E-mail: **kasey@qai-inc.com**

SBDFG—Society for Bio-Dynamic Farming and Gardening in Ontario
RR #2, Elora, Ontario N0B 1S0
Phone : (519) 843-6822
E-mail: **mailbox@biodynamics.on.ca**
The B.D. Society certifies growers according the their standards using
the certification mark "Demeter" on their products.

SOURCES OF INFORMATION

COG—Canadian Organic Growers Inc.
Toll-free: 1-888-375-7383
Fax: (613) 236-0743
Internet: **http://www.cog.ca**

EAP—Ecological Agriculture Project
Internet: **http://www.eap.mcgill.ca**

EFAO—Ecological Farmers Association of Ontario
Phone: (519) 822-8606
Internet: **http://www.efao.ca**

OMAFRA—Ontario Ministry of Agriculture, Food and Rural Affairs
Internet: **http://www.gov.on.ca/OMAFRA/**
Martin, Hugh. Organic Farming in Ontario Factsheet Order # 98-029, a
publication provided by the Ministry of Agriculture, Food and Rural
Affairs, June 1998.

FOOD AND NUTRITION

GENETICALLY ENGINEERED AGRIBUSINESS—PANDORA'S BOX?

GMO (genetically modified organisms), GM (genetically modified), biotech foods, frankenfoods, terminator seeds. Almost thirty years old, genetic engineering (GE) has led to cross-breeding of different species (not known in nature). This means inserting the genetic material of the DNA from plants, animals, insects, soil micro-organisms, bacteria, viruses or humans into other plants or animals in order to develop certain desired characteristics such as: resistance to certain pests, an increased tolerance for larger amounts of pesticides, bigger or faster growth, change in texture of the final product or ability to grow in an environment in which it is not usually found.

Some examples are strawberries with arctic char genes, human genes in pigs, Bt bacterium inserted into corn, potato with jellyfish genes to glow when they need to be watered, super GE-enhanced salmon—twice as large as any salmon in history—vegetables with scorpion genes, tomato with flounder genes, GE cows that produce milk similar to human breast milk. The potential of this sort of inventive creation is appalling.

Too much about it is unpredictable. GMOs will themselves evolve, interact with other organisms and mutate. They can be neither recalled nor contained. There has been little scientific study about the short- or long-term health risks from GE crops and food. Many would agree that this is worrisome, to say the least!

Canadian geneticist and environmentalist David Suzuki at a Toronto conference in 2001 stated directly, "When industry (scientists) say these products are safe, they are either stupid or lying." It may be that they are both.

Biotech companies (often now merged with pharmaceutical ones), such as Syngenta (Novartis, AstraZeneca), Monsanto (Pharmacia), Dupont also gave us Agent Orange, toxic pesticides, toxic waste, silicon implants, aspartame, etc. These industries' science is top secret and often deceptive in regards to product safety.

Agricultural scientist Prof. Ann Clark of Guelph University, who has written extensively about the risk of genetic engineering, points out that in their haste to develop GE crops, researchers either completely neglected or ignored considering information from other scientific disciplines such as:

- Entomology: e.g., insects can develop complete pesticide resistance in one single generation
- Agronomy: e.g., sudden unexpected magnesium depletion in food crops impact on human physiology
- Virology: e.g., GE crops promote the evolution of new viruses against which no defence exists
- Evolutionary Genetics: e.g., large crop failures of soy, cotton and some potato because altered genes diminished their ability to adapt to sudden weather changes.

From a global perspective, GE crops are detrimental to human health because they:

- have greater requirement for water (lowering water tables and stressing the world water supply even more)
- speed up evolution of pesticide-resistant bugs (there are now more than 600 totally resistant pests, compared to 6 in 1947)
- increase the need for pesticides
- produce super weeds through cross-breeding with wild plants
- degrade the soil
- kill useful pollinators and beneficial bacteria
- decrease crops' nutritional value
- cause resistance of dangerous bacteria to antibiotics.

Some of the first research done on GE potatoes was carried out by Prof. Arpad Pusztai of the Rowett Institute of Scotland, who promptly lost his job after publicly stating he would not eat GE foods due to insufficient testing procedures. He has since become outspoken on the topic of GM safety.

His controversial research indicated that after thirty days of feeding on GE potatoes, rats showed:

- Immune disruption (immunosuppression, decreased thymus function)
- Hormonal problems

FOOD AND NUTRITION

- Retarded brain growth
- Gastrointestinal inflammation

His studies resulted in an indefinite moratorium by the European Union on all GE foods. Most of the world's countries and Europe have banned GE foods, except for the GE-producing USA and Canada. This is happening despite various polls showing, for instance, that 94% of Canadians would prefer to avoid GE foods and 70% want GE foods clearly labelled.

Canadian and US regulatory agencies have approved the following GM foods:

- Canola
- Corn (sweet and for popcorn)
- Cotton
- Flax
- Potato
- Soybean
- Squash
- Sugar beet
- Tomato

All US dairy products are allowed to contain bovine growth hormone (GE).

In additon, there are a number of GE ingredients that find their way into various foods such as:

- Aspartame (Nutrasweet), which gets into 9000 products on the market (and is a dangerous product in itself aside from the GE factor)
- Baker's yeast
- Brewer's yeast
- Riboflavin (B2)
- Alpha amylase
- Hemicellulase
- Lipase and Triaclyglycerol

Some vitamins may have GE content. You can call the 1-800 listed on most containers to ask about this.

All "junk food" contains GE products. The majority of the North American food industry uses GE foods, although some companies have recently declared that they are or will be using GE-free products (e.g., Gerber's, McCain's, Frito-Lay). However, why, if Kellog's, Nestle, Heinz, Enfamil and Similac can promise to produce GE-free food for Europe, can't they do the same for North America?

Farmers speaking to agricultural journalist Steven Sprinkel, writing for *Acres USA* (Sept. 18, 1999), noted that animals refuse to eat GE corn or soybeans. "What is it that they know instinctively that we ignore?" Since we have apparently lost these self-preserving instincts, we should use our intellects to reject poorly researched GE foods and—

- Buy organic
- Ask our local grocery manager to carry GE-free products
- Write food industry companies demanding GE-free food
- Write our government representatives demanding GE-free food or at least adequate labeling for informed choice
- Become educated, become concerned and become active.

THE LABEL GAME

Governing bodies

Consumer and Corporate Affairs Canada
(Food and Drugs Act and Regulations)
(Consumer Packaging and Labeling Act and Regulations)
"Ingredients must be listed in descending order of weight"
- with the exception of the following, which can appear at the end of the ingredient list in any order:
  - spices, seasoning, herbs (except salt), natural & artificial flavours, flavour enhancers, food additives, vitamins, minerals and their salts
- specific ingredients may change week to week, e.g., may contain coconut oil, soy oil, corn oil.

FOOD AND NUTRITION

The following items are not required to appear on the label
- mineral oil used to grease pans
- additives occurring unintentionally e.g., pesticide residue
- chemicals from packaging
- ingredients of ingredients, e.g., the constituents of margarine in a cake
- **GE food**, on its own or as an ingredient

The following require no ingredient list
- bulk foods packaged by the retailer
- products baked on the premises
- meat and poultry cooked on the premises
- alcohol, vinegar
- individually portioned foods, e.g., mustard
- vending machine and coffee truck foods
- "one-bite" candies

If you have allergies or sensitivities, be sure to **READ THE LABEL**. A good rule is that if the product contains too many chemicals or names you can't pronounce, then **don't buy it**!

GRAINS

These are the seed of the plant. They are high in carbohydrates, fibre, trace minerals, and B vitamins. They can provide a good source of protein when combined with seeds/nuts, legumes, or dairy products (see page 140 regarding complementary proteins).

FOOD AND NUTRITION

ANATOMY OF A GRAIN

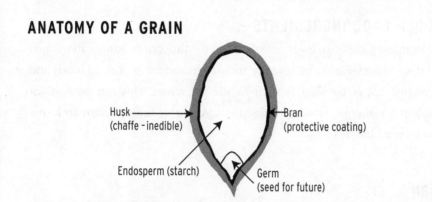

Husk ——— (chaffe – inedible)

Bran (protective coating)

Endosperm (starch)

Germ (seed for future)

FAMILY	FAMILY MEMBER	
GRAINS		
Grass Family	**Gluten free**	**Gluten containing**
	• corn	• barley
	• millet	• rye
	• rice	• spelt
	• wild rice	• wheat
	• teff	• oats
	• sorghum	• kamut
		• triticale

NON-GRAIN ALTERATIVES

Goosefoot family	Quinoa
Amaranth family	Amaranth
Buckwheat family	Buckwheat
Spurge family	Cassava, mandioca, tapioca
Arum	Arrowroot–many different kinds
Banana	
Canna	
Arrowroot	

HIDDEN FOOD INGREDIENTS

The next few pages give information about the most commonly eaten foods and their hidden forms, i.e., as they are used in various processed foods and forms but not recognized as such by the consumer. This can be a major problem for allergic/sensitive individuals. **Again, it is important to know how to read labels.**

CORN

Corn is a major allergen for many individuals. It is a hidden ingredient in most factory-produced foods.

Forms of Corn

corn cereals	corn sugars	parched corn
corn flour	corn syrups	popcorn
corn meal	grits	vegetable oil
corn oil	hominy	
corn starch	maize	
fresh corn	canned corn	corn fritters
frozen corn	roasting ears	succotash

Names appearing on ingredient labels

Cartose	Cerlose	Corn sugar	Corn starch
Corn syrup	Dextrin	Dextrose	Dyno
Fructose	Glucose	Dextrimaltose	Kremel
Maize	Maltose	Malt	Manitol
Hydrolyzed vegetable oil	Puretose	Sorbitol	Sweetose

Common Contacts

- paper cups, cartons, envelopes, stamps (corn starch)
- some coughdrops, syrup, pills, tablets, suppositories, ointments
- some corn-based vitamin and mineral supplements

- most alcoholic beverages
- adhesives
- toothpastes, mouthwashes
- bath and body powders, starch for ironing clothing

Some categories of food that could contain corn

bacon	frying batters	preserves
baking, commercial	graham crackers	puddings
baking mixes	gravy	succotash
baking powder	hominy grits	starch
beer	hams	salad dressing
cakes	Harvard beets	sauces
candy	icing sugar	sausages
carbonated	icing	spaghetti
beverages	ice creams	sugar—glucose,
cereals	jams & jellies	fructose & dextrose
cereal flakes	jello	syrup
corn, fresh	ketchup	sherbet
chili	leavening agents	soup
Chinese food	liquor	soy milks
coffee, instant	luncheon meats	shortening
cookies	meal	salt
cream pie fillings	margarine	tea, instant
chewing gum	MSG	tortilla
dates	noodles	vanillin
dietetic mixes	oil	vinegar
eggnog	popcorn	vegetables,
fritters	pastry	processed
flour, bleached	peanut butter	vegetable oils
fish, processed	pickles	waffles
fried food	pizza	wines
fruits, processed	pork & beans	yogurt

Fortunately there are many corn free products on the market. When you do your shopping, read the labels and ask questions. Of course, if you make the product yourself, you can easily cut out the corn.

Unfortunately, today, most of our corn is genetically modified, and regrettably it is not labelled as such; therefore, do you really know what you are eating?

WHEAT
Wheat is also a common food allergen, and once again is found in many forms and foods.

Forms of Wheat
flour
starch—the carbohydrate minus the wheat protein
gluten—the major protein in wheat in isolated form
berry—the seed
cracked wheat/bulgar (cracked, partially cooked, toasted)
wheat germ
wheat grass
couscous—ground semolina wheat, precooked
wheat flakes

Names appearing on ingredient labels

wheat	wheat starch
whole wheat	wheat germ
enriched flour	cracked wheat flour
flour	farina
malt	durham flour

Graham flour—coarse type of whole wheat
semolina—durham wheat flour with the bran and germ removed MSG
    (monosodium glutamate can be wheat or beet derived) HVP (hydrolyzed
    vegetable protein) HPP (hydrolyzed plant protein)
TVP (textured vegetable protein)

Common Contacts

- prepared foods; as a thickening agent/flour and as a filler e.g., luncheon meats, hotdogs, casseroles, sausages, hamburger mix
- cereal fillers, cold cereals
- noodles/pasta, couscous
- cheese spread
- drinks with malt, malted milk, Ovaltine, Postum
- commercially prepared baked goods e.g., biscuits, crackers, pretzels, rolls, breads, (even rye, soy, corn, pumpernickel and other breads may contain wheat)
- some buckwheat noodles and pancake mixes, croutons
- zwieback
- bouillon cubes
- ice cream, candy
- baking powder
- thickened salad dressings and sauces, including mayonnaise
- white vinegar
- some alcoholic beverages
- meats dredged in flour before cooking
- dumplings

ALTERNATIVES TO WHEAT FLOUR

Wheat contains a high amount of gluten, an elastic protein that is responsible for the distinct characteristics of wheat bread. Alternatives will have their own special qualities. After some experimentation, you will know which substitutes work best in various recipes. Please keep in mind that each individual's sensitivities are unique, and any substitutes must be tested for tolerance. Also, individuals who are gluten-sensitive will not be able to tolerate any form of grain containing gluten.

FOOD AND NUTRITION

Replace 1 cup white or whole wheat flour with:

GRAIN/NON-GRAIN	1 CUP WHEAT FLOUR =
Amaranth	1 cup amaranth, $1/4$ cup amaranth + $3/4$ cup rice
	$3/4$ cup amaranth + $1/4$ cup arrowroot, tapioca or potato
Arrowroot	$1/2$ cup
Barley	$1/2$ to 1 cup
Bean flour	$3/4$ cup
Buckwheat	$3/4$ cup
Chick Pea	$1/2$ to $3/4$ cup
Corn meal, Corn flour	1 cup fine cornmeal or $7/8$ to 1 cup corn flour
Corn starch	$1/2$ to $3/4$ cup
Kamut	1 cup
Millet	1 cup
Oat flour	$7/8$ cup to $1\frac{1}{2}$ cup
Potato flour	$1/3$ cup potato four & $2/3$ cup rye flour, $1/2$ cup potato flour and $1/2$ cup soy flour
Rice flour	$3/4$ cup to $7/8$ cup, $5/8$ cup rice flour and $1/3$ cup rye flour
Rye	$3/4$ to 1 cup, $1/2$ cup rye flour and $1/2$ cup oat flour
Soy	$3/4$ to $7/8$ cup
Spelt	1 cup

Substitute Thickeners

- Starches—arrowroot, potato, tapioca
- Flours—see above list
- Vegetable—cooked puree of starchy vegetable or shredded raw starch vegetable
- Nuts—ground

Breadcrumb Substitutes

- Rice cereal, rice cakes, rye crackers, oat crackers, potato chips
- Dried rye bread/essene bread—grated
- Alternative flours, oatmeal
- Grated, starchy vegetable
- Ground nuts

FOOD AND NUTRITION

SOY

Soy is a member of the legume family. It is an excellent protein when combined with grains, seeds, or dairy products. It is low in fat, and high in carbohydrates and fibre. Its versatility and nutritional value have made it a standard in many eastern cuisines. In North America it is used frequently in processed foods and is becoming a common food allergen. Soy may also be encountered in non-food items and unfortunately is often a GE food (see page 154.)

Forms

- Flour
- Tofu—the bean is washed, soaked, ground and boiled. A coagulant is added to the resulting milk and the curd is formed into squares. Consistency ranges from soft to firm.
- Oil
- Bean
- Grits—TVP: (Textured Vegetable Protein)—highly processed to provide a protein source resembling meat products
- Milk—soy milk, baby formula
- Miso—soy cheese: no lactose or cholesterol, but it does contain calcium caseinate (milk derived protein)
- Tempeh
- Soy sauce

Common Contacts

Baked goods
Cereals
Meats
Milk substitutes
Ice cream
Ice cream substitutes
Sauces
Salad dressings

Celluloid
Linoleum
Adhesives
Nitroglycerine
Automobile parts
Massage creams
Paper sizing
Paper finishes

FOOD AND NUTRITION

Candies (including carob chips)   Cloth, blankets
Soups   Fertilizer
Butter substitutes   Glycerin
Custards   Varnish, paints
Printing inks   Candles

DAIRY PRODUCTS

COW'S MILK

Milk is another of North America's common food allergens, and once again it is a hidden ingredient in many processed and restaurant foods. Some individuals get sick from milk because they cannot digest the sugar it contains; this is called lactose intolerance. Others cannot tolerate the milk protein and, although symptoms may be similar, this is classified as a milk allergy or sensitivity.

Forms

- Whole   (3.25% fat with a cream line)
- Homogenized   (3.25% fat with no cream line)
- 2 percent   (2% fat)
- 1 percent   (1% fat)
- Skim   (less than 0.5% fat)
- Evaporated   (7.5% fat)
- Sweetened condensed   (8.5% fat)
- Dry milk
- Creams, sour cream
- Devonshire   (clotted cream)
- Filled milk   (dry milk, soy, vegetable or coconut oil)
- Yogurt   (milk plus friendly bacteria)
- Sour milk   (lactic acid plus whole or skim milk)
- Buttermilk   (skim milk plus bacterial culture)

FOOD AND NUTRITION

- Butter   (80% fat plus water plus milk solids)
- Clarified butter (Ghee)   (water and milk solids removed)
- Cheeses

Names appearing on ingredient labels

- Casein (milk protein)   Lactose (milk sugar)   Curds
- Lactate   Calcium Caseinate   Caseinate
- Lactalbumin   Lactoglobulin   Milk Solids
- Sodium Caseinate   Whey (milk protein)

Common Contacts

- Baked goods, breads, cookies, crackers
- Cream desserts, including ice cream and some sherbets
- Creamed soups, sauces and vegetables
- Boiled salad dressings
- Factory-made candies, with the exception of hard candy
- Chocolate/cocoa drinks, carob chips
- Ovaltine and malted drinks
- Many egg dishes
- Scalloped, au gratin, and mashed dishes (e.g., potato)
- Foods fried in butter
- Processed meats

FOOD AND NUTRITION

Note: If milk comes from the USA, it will contain Bovine Growth Hormone unless it is organic. Milk additives are present in some non-dairy products such as margarine, so be sure to read labels.

Dairy products are easy to eat and provide a good source of nutrients (protein, calcium), however, their value can be overestimated. Humans are the only animals who continue to consume milk after being weaned. Two-thirds of the world's population lacks the lactase enzyme, and milk consumption for these people can cause a severe problem due to lactose intolerance. Milk can also be a major sensitizer in utero for a susceptible fetus. Later on, it can be a major allergen causing many newborn and childhood problems such as upper respiratory and ear infections and other allergy related problems. Recently, milk consumption has been implicated in early onset diabetes mellitus.

GOAT'S MILK

Some individuals who cannot tolerate cow's milk can drink goat's milk with no difficulty. The differences are as follows:

- Both milks contain lactose (milk sugar).
- Both milks contain the protein casein.
- Goat's milk contains whey, a protein that differs from that in cow's milk.
- The fat globules are smaller in goat's milk and therefore easier to digest.
- The calcium content in goat's milk is higher.
- The folacin (folic acid) content in goat's milk is lower.

YOGURT

Cow's or goat's milk

Friendly bacteria
(Lactobacillus bulgaricus
and Lactobacillus acidophilus
are the most commonly used)

Lactic acid and
breakdown of milk,
sugar, protein and fat

FOOD AND NUTRITION

Kefir

Kefir is a fermented milk, which contains a blend of cultures including Saccharomyces kefir, Torula kefir, Lactobacillus caucasus, Streptococcus lactis, and other organisms. It can be made from cow, soy, goat and sheep's milk.

Cheese

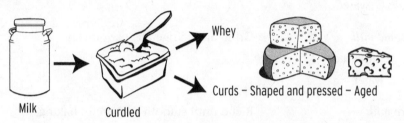

Milk   Curdled   Whey   Curds – Shaped and pressed – Aged

All cheese, with the exception of cottage cheese, contains mold. All cheese contains tyramine. This substance is also found in chocolate, yogurt, red wine, gin, rye, and vodka. It can trigger migraine.

Alternatives to Dairy Products
Milks

Soy milk
1 C. soy flour + 4 C. water

Let mixture sit for 2 hours, bring to a boil and simmer 20 min. Cool and strain, sweeten to taste.

Cashew milk
½ C. raw cashews +
1 C. water + 1 t. honey

Grind nuts until pasty, blend with water until smooth, then add honey and vanilla.

Almond milk
5 T. blanched almonds +
1 C. water + 1 t. honey

Blend ingredients until smooth.

Coconut milk
1 C. unsweetened shredded coconut + 2 C. water

Strain through cheese cloth. Soak coconut in water, blend and strain through cheese cloth.

Nut milk ½ C. nuts + 1C. liquid	Soak overnight, blend to a paste and add liquid to desired consistency.
Sunflower Seed Milk white 1C. sunflower seeds + 3½ C. water	Soak overnight, blend until a milk is produced. Strain.
Sesame milk 1C. sesame seeds + 1⅜C. water	Grind and refrigerate, use quickly.
Rice milk 1C. cooked brown rice + 1–3 C. water	Blend until smooth and use in baking, desserts, etc.

Filtered or spring water
Vegetable cooking water
Fruit juice and Fruit puree
Goat's milk

Many of these milks can be found today as commercially prepared products in your local health food store and even your local grocery store. Just be sure to read the label, so that you can make a wise choice.

Butter
- Nut butters (peanut, cashew, hazelnut, sesame, tahini, sunflower, etc.)
- Soy butter (check the label for ingredients)
- Pureed fruit
- Avocado paste
- Sweet potato, mashed
- Fruit-sweetened fruit spread (available at health food stores)

In baking:

vegetable oils   ⅔ C. oil = 1C. solid fat reduce other liquids
                  and bake slightly longer at a lower temperature

animal fats   1C. lard (organic source)

nut butters   use in the same proportions as a soft butter

SWEETENERS

All sweeteners are carbohydrates and, as such, they are made up of carbon, hydrogen, and oxygen. The means by which these elements are connected defines the form of carbohydrates; cellulose, complex carbohydrates, simple sugars (monosaccharides), or double sugars (disaccharides). All carbohydrates, with the exception of cellulose, are converted into glucose (blood sugar) during the digestive process. Glucose provides the body with energy. This energy is most readily available from the sugars. Starches (complex carbohydrates) must be broken into sugars before they can be transformed into glucose; a cellulose is not digested, but provides bulk for the effective functioning of the digestive tract (see page 137).

Most sugars are derived from cane sugar. Historical data show that in England in 1815, a person consumed an average of 15 pounds of refined sugar per year. By 1955, this figure had risen to 120 pounds/year per person. In Canada, the average refined sugar consumption is close to 180 pounds/year, per person.

The refining process of sugar (making it white), removes 93% of the chromium, 89% of manganese, 98% of cobalt, 83% of copper, 98% of zinc and 98% of the magnesium that is contained in raw sugar. All of these minerals are essential for life.

Forms

Granules, crystals, powder, in foods and syrups.

• White table sugar: from sugar cane or sugar beets; highly refined.

FOOD AND NUTRITION

- Raw sugar: this is white sugar before the refining process. Unless it is organic, it contains various contaminants.
- Turbinado sugar: this goes through all refining steps of white sugar, with the exception of the removal of molasses.
- Brown sugar: white sugar plus molasses
- Molasses: a by-product of cane sugar refining. It is high in minerals, but contains chemical residue.
- Barbados/unsulphured molasses: processing of sugar with the express purpose of making molasses.
- Sorghum molasses: syrup from the juice of the sorghum plant (a grain).
- Cane sugar syrup: similar to Barbados molasses.
- Maple syrup/sugar
- Sucanat: from dried granulated whole cane juice. Only the water is removed.
- Fructose: can be produced through the chemical splitting of sucrose into glucose and fructose, or the conversion of corn syrup starches. This sugar is 60% sweeter than white table sugar.
- Glucose: Corn syrup
- Honey: Nectar (containing sucrose) is refined by the bee into fructose + glucose + water + sucrose. 20 to 60% sweeter than white sugar. The flavour depends on the flower source. Do not feed to children less than one year, as it can transmit botulism.
- Barley malt syrup: Can be 100% barley or a combination of barley and corn. 40 to 70% as sweet as white sugar.
- Rice syrup/rice malt syrup: maltose (45%) + glucose (3%) + complex carbohydrates (50%)
- Amasake: rice sweetener. Cultured brown rice is added to cooked rice. Starch is changed into maltose + glucose.
- Date sugar: ground, dehydrated dates. Almost as sweet as white sugar.
- Fruit juice: concentrates can reach up to 66% of the sweetness of white sugar.

- Stevia: a herb that is very sweet. It has no effect on blood sugar and contains no calories. Can be baked or cooked at any temperature without breaking down.
- Sugar alcohols:
  Mannitol—from corn glucose can reach up to 65% of the sweetness of white sugar
  Sorbitol—also from corn glucose, and almost as sweet as mannitol; has a slow rate of absorption and may cause diarrhea
  Xylitol—from birchwood chips

Artificial sweeteners such as aspartame, saccharin, sodium cyclamate, sorbitol, Twink etc. are not recommended, especially for chemically sensitive individuals and children because of the negative heath effects associated with them.

Aspartame is marketed under the popular names of NutraSweet™, Equal™, Spoonful™, and Equal-measure™, and is found as an ingredient in many "sugar-free" candies, gum and diet soft drinks. Aspartame is composed of three chemicals—aspartic acid, phenylalanine and methanol. Methanol makes up 10% of aspartame and is also known as **wood alcohol —a deadly poison.** When aspartame is heated above 86 degrees Fahrenheit, free methanol is created. This can easily occur with improper storage of any food or beverage product containing aspartame, or when these food products are heated. When ingested, aspartame breaks down into three amino acids, as well as methanol. The continuing digestive process then converts this **methanol into formaldehyde.** Aspartame has been declared by some to be the most dangerous food additive on the market, and some place it in the category of a "chemical poison." A few of the conditions that have been linked to excessive aspartic excitation include: multiple sclerosis, amyotrophic lateral sclerosis (ALS), memory loss, hormonal imbalance, hearing loss, epilepsy, Alzheimer's disease, Parkinson's disease, hypoglycemia, AIDS dementia, brain lesions and neuro-endocrine problems. Even illnesses such as those incurred by Desert Storm troops have been associated with aspartame ingestion. They were provided aspartame beverages, which, due to the desert conditions, were heated to over 86 degrees. The troops returned home experiencing symptoms mimicking those associated with chemical poisoning by formaldehyde.

YEAST

Yeasts are one-celled plants that are members of the fungus family. In one pound of yeast, there are 3200 billion unique cells. Yeast will grow in the presence of any sugar and give off alcohol and carbon dioxide.

Forms of Yeast

Baker's Yeast
- Used for leavening bread, and found in many forms
- Active dry yeast—yeast that has been freeze-dried to retain its activity
- Instant or quick-rise yeasts—leaven bread more rapidly than active dry yeast although not recommended for most of the non-wheat bread machine breads

Brewer's Yeast
- Contained in alcoholic beverages such as beer

Wild Yeast
- Leavens bread much more slowly than baker's yeast
- This yeast is a different strain than commercial baker's yeast
- Used in the production of sourdough cultures (see section on sourdough, p. 176)

Nutritional Yeast
- Dried yeast used as a natural source of protein and B-complex vitamins

Common Contacts

- Alcoholic beverages (see page 100–101)
- Black tea leaves
- Nutritional supplements
- Smoked foods
- Vinegar (grain or fruit + sugar + yeast)
- Products containing vinegar: mayonnaise, salad dressing, mustard, ketchup, sauces (worcestershire, steak, barbecue, chili, shrimp, pickles, pickled foods, relishes, olives)
- Malt (fermented from corn, wheat or barley)
- Miso, tempheh
- Baked goods, e.g., breads, raised doughnuts, crackers, coffee cakes
- Enriched flour
- Milk fortified with yeast
- Citric acid a) lemon or pineapple juice + one of the fungus family
  b) fermented corn, sugar beets, or molasses.

Note: For individuals with mold sensitivities and/or yeast problems, controlling the intake of certain foods is essential for improvement. There are many versions of the yeast-free diet, some more restrictive than others. Should your doctor recommend such a diet for you, please refer to the section on Candida management (pp. 69 and 230).

Alternative Leaveners

Baking powder: Generally, premixed powders contain corn or wheat. To avoid these contacts, make your own.

a) $\frac{1}{2}$ tsp. cream of tartar + $\frac{1}{4}$ tsp. baking soda

b) $\frac{3}{4}$ C. cream of tartar + 9 Tbsp. baking soda + 6 Tbsp. potato starch

c) 2 parts arrowroot starch + 1 part baking soda + 1 part cream of tartar

To replace 2 tsp. of baking powder, include ½ tsp. baking soda and 1 cup of an acidic ingredient such as: sour cream, milk, applesauce, mashed banana, or yogurt. Other recipes will use varying amounts of baking soda and unbuffered vitamin C powder.

Sourdough

Sourdough breads are yeast breads that are leavened by a sourdough starter, or culture, rather than by commercial baker's yeast. Sourdough cultures contain wild yeast and bacteria of the genus lactobacillus that work together in a symbiotic relationship. The wild yeast produces gas, which in turn causes the bread to rise, and the bacteria gives the bread its sour flavour. Some individuals who are allergic to commercial baker's yeast will tolerate sourdough breads, and this may be because they are not allergic to wild yeast.

Sourdough cultures are most often started with wheat flour, but as it is fed with an alternative flour and transferred many times in the process of activating it, the wheat flour is diluted out.

Be sure to read the label of any sourdough bread you propose to buy, after, of course, checking with your environmental physician regarding your individual sensitivities and considering his or her advice on your tolerance.

EGGS

Many individuals are allergic/sensitive to eggs. Frequently, the egg white is the problem, although it is possible to be sensitive to the egg yolk as well. In addition, the cooking method may make a difference. Eggs are a perfect and most nutritionally balanced food with all necessary nutrients, able to support the embryo and developing chick. Contrary to common belief, although eggs contain a lot of cholesterol, they actually lower cholesterol when eaten due to their high content of lecithin and omega-3 essential fatty acids (EFA). **Only organic eggs** are able to yield a high level of omega-3 EFAs. Fumigation of hen-laying coops with flea-killing pesticides which penetrate the porous structure of eggshells, dramatically decreases the omega-3 EFAs.

Forms

Egg white   Dried egg
Egg yolk   Meringue
Egg yolk solids   Powdered eggs
Whole egg

NAMES APPEARING ON INGREDIENT LABELS

Vitellin   Ovovitellin
Albumin   Livetin
Ovomucin   Ovomucoid

Common contacts

Puddings, custards   Marshmallows
Baked goods   Meringue
Mayonnaise   Boullion, consommé
Soufflés   Egg drop and noodle soup
Binder in meat dishes   Pasta
Some cheese mixes   Sauces e.g., mayonnaise, tartar,
                              Hollandaise
Ice cream, sherbet   Vaccines derived from eggs
Regular baking powder   Dessert powders
Batter for deep fat frying French toast, pancakes, waffles
Prepared foods   Malted milk drinks
Icing

Alternatives to Chicken Eggs

- duck, turkey, or goose eggs
- 1 tbsp. flaxseed powder + 3 tbsp. water—boil until thickens slightly
- starchy vegetables (great with meats)
- 2 tbsp. fruit puree (works well in cookies)
- ½ tsp. baking powder + 2 tbsp. flour + ½ tbsp. fat.

FOOD AND NUTRITION

- 2 tbsp. water + 2 tsp. baking powder
- for egg yolk replacement use ½ tsp. baking powder + 2 tbsp. flour
- for one egg white replacement use 1 tsp. gelatin, 3 tbsp. cold water and 7 tsp. boiling water
- for meringue replacement use 5 tbsp. ground flaxseed and 5 cups of cold water; soak together for 1 hour, then simmer for 20 minutes; Strain and refrigerate, and beat as you would egg whites.

PORK

Forms

Fresh	Cured	Processed
Roast, sausage,	Bacon & drippings,	Wieners, Vienna
Chops, liver	Pork & beans,	sausage
Kidney, cracklings	Ham, bacon bits,	Luncheon meats
Chitterlings	Pickled pig's feet,	mincemeat, Spam
Souse (head cheese)	Salt pork	Liverwurst

Common Contacts

Lard & shortening	Margarine	Vegetable stock
Instant foods	Mayonnaise	Fried foods
Non-dairy creamer	Mexican food	Chinese food
Polynesian food	Potato chips	Candy bars
Ice cream	Gelatin, jello	Bakery products
Glycerin products	Some drugs	Glue

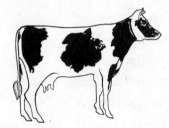

BEEF

Forms

Fresh beef cuts	Veal (baby beef)	Gelatin
Corned beef	Pastrami	Sausage
Liverwurst	Sandwich meats	Wieners
Soups: Consommé	Glue used in drink	
Bouillon	cartons and labels	

Note: *Liver can come from any animal; beef, calf, pork, lamb, and chicken are the most common.*

One of the liver's key functions is to remove waste products ingested along with foods (e.g., pesticides). Consequently, if liver is eaten, be sure to use an organic source.

FLAXSEED

- The seed of the flax plant; it is also known as linseed.

Forms

- fabric—linen, damask, cambric, thread, toweling, oil cloth, art linen...
- food —oil (linseed/flaxseed*), flour, seed

Common contacts

- Cereals (e.g., Red River)
- Some cough remedies
- Fodder for cattle and poultry
- Hair setting lotions (e.g., Kremel)

- Furniture polish
- Carron oil, linseed oil
- Paints and varnishes
- Linoleum (and linoleum dust)
- Printer's and lithographic ink
- Soft soap
- Some depilatories
- Egg replacer
- Insulation (Bi-flax, Flaxlinum)
- Rugs, straw mats
- Wax paper
- Furniture stuffing
- Fibre board

Never cook with or heat flaxseed/linseed oil for human consumption because it is poisonous in its heated form.

Cold flaxseed oil is perfectly safe to ingest and is used for many chronic, degenerative and inflammatory conditions. It is an excellent supply of omega-3 essential fatty acids that are physiologically more effective in combination with omega-6 fatty acids, usually in a ratio of 1:2.

FOOD AND NUTRITION

Management

GENERAL MANAGEMENT CONCEPTS

The most effective treatment is to prevent the development of body overload. If overload has already occurred, attention must be paid to reducing the stress factors. In both cases, this involves careful management of all aspects contributing to the individual's illness. The environmentally sensitive individual can exercise control over his/her sensitivities by:

- Developing greater awareness of the problems: how you react, what the problem involves, where problems can be encountered.
- Learning to avoid the trigger: complete avoidance is best, but even partial avoidance helps decrease the load.
- Developing a repertoire of coping tactics: for example, take a walk in the fresh air after attending a meeting where people smoked; put an air filter into your home or place of work.
- Taking prescribed treatment extracts / medications / supplements.
- Improving the nutrition of the individual and family.
- Detoxification using hydrotherapy, nutritional supplements.
- Changing attitudes towards the environment, understanding the unity between the environment and ourselves.

Attitude

"When the going gets tough, the tough get going."

Environmental illness does not disappear, but it can be brought under control. Recognition and understanding is the first step towards making positive change, but this must be followed by constructive action.

Pacing

"Slow and steady wins the race."

It took time to reach a state of overload, and reversal of the process does not occur overnight. In fact, tackling changes too quickly can create additional stress and cause the individual to give up on the very measures that will make a difference in the long term. Set goals and work towards them.

Balance and Moderation

"All things in moderation."

It is impossible to eliminate all problem items from our lives. By modifying areas within our control, we can decrease our total body load, making it easier to balance the remaining weight. Do the best you can to effect change, keep your goals in sight, and remember; "all things in moderation."

Individuality

"What works for one may not work for another."

Remember, we are all individual. Our total body load is unique and so are the reactions we have. Keep this in mind as you read through the following chapter on management techniques. Never forget to test a new product, food, or idea for your own tolerance.

Interrelationships

Keep in mind that environmental illness is complex, resulting from the interrelationship of many separate elements, the combination of which leads to

MANAGEMENT

an overburdened body. Management must be directed at all problem areas, the goal being to decrease total body load.

Methods of Management

Like the overload picture, management of overload is unique for each individual. There are, however, certain key techniques that can be utilized by most people to reduce their overload.

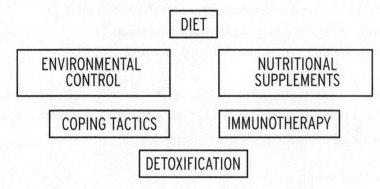

The following pages outline some of the basic coping tactics. Most are a matter of common sense, but when we are faced with situations which sometimes seem impossible, a combination of these tactics can be just what we are looking for. The problem may not disappear, but the situation becomes much more manageable.

Increase Awareness

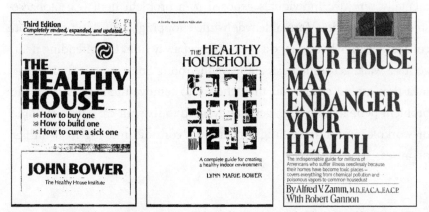

Source: The Healthy House Institute, 430 North Service Road, Bloomington, IN 47408

The first step towards improving a situation is to find out more about it. **Education is very important.** Specifically:

- What are the sources of your total body load?
- Where and how do you come into contact with them?
- How do you react to them?
- What can be done to avoid them?
- What is Clinical Ecology/Environmental Illness?
- What can be done to decrease environmental pollution?
- Start to see yourself as a part of your environment.
- See the environment as your life support system.

In the long term, it also helps to increase the awareness of others: your family and friends, your child's teacher, the people you work with. Please refer to the bibliography at the end of this book.

Remove the Problem

Inspect your home thoroughly. It is preferable to get rid of the problem completely, but if this is not possible, at least remove it from your immediate living environment.

Remove Yourself from the Problem

Have you ever thought "I'll just make it through this meeting, (grocery list, car repair) and then I'll go home and relax?" If you are like many environmentally sensitive individuals exposed to a problem item (e.g., tobacco smoke at a meeting, formaldehyde while shopping), you don't relax, you collapse. Learn when to take a break and get away from the offending item, go for a walk, get some fresh air, leave the room. Some people find stricter measures are necessary and they choose to remove themselves from the problem permanently (e.g., get a body shop to fix your car). If your home or workplace or surroundings are unsafe, consider moving to healthier premises.

MANAGEMENT

Use Safe/Environmentally Friendly Products

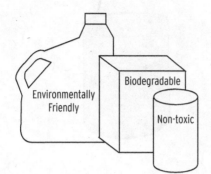

With increased awareness of the environment and health, there are more and more alternatives on the market every day. Remember, each individual's sensitivities vary, so test a product for your own tolerance. Choose non-perfumed, dye-free, phosphate-free, non-toxic products.

Clean It

Get rid of the mold and dust, using tolerated cleaning products. Don't forget to keep your ventilation, filtration and humidification systems clean too. Have your ducts cleaned professionally, occasionally. When planning your home environment, keep ease of cleaning in mind. Avoid clutter, furnish the rooms according to the principles of Feng Shui. (*The Complete Illustrated Guide to Feng Shui* by Lillian Too, Element Books Ltd., 1996).

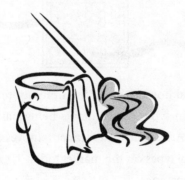

MANAGEMENT

Seal It

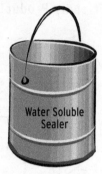

e.g., steel cabinets

Mattress cover—cotton and/or special anti-mite cover

If you can't get rid of the problem item, look at the way you are storing it. Perfumes, paint, thinners, glues, synthetics and so on, all off-gas, even with the lids on. Either get rid of them or seal them well and store in an airtight box. Also be aware of potential mold growth in storage areas. Keep boxes and wood off the floor, and don't forget to clean. For example, pressboard located under sinks, desks, shelving, etc., can be sealed with a water soluble sealer that will provide a hard coating that prevents future out-gassing.

Filter the Air

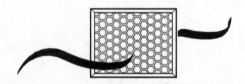

The air inside a typical home is up to five times more polluted than the air outside; the two main types of pollutants being particulates and volatile organic compounds. An effective air cleaner removes both particulates and VOCs. There are many types on the market today. Therefore, it is important to be an informed consumer.

Electronic Air Cleaners

- High voltage is used to electrically charge particles so that they may be attracted to a series of charged metal plates
- Efficiency declines rapidly with use, leaving an average efficiency of only 50%
- Requires frequent cleaning to maintain efficiency
- Emits undesirable ozone (O_3) as a by-product.

Ionizing Air Cleaners/Electrostatic Air Cleaners

- Dust particles are electrically charged and attracted to the unit
- Emit ozone (O_3) as a by-product

HEPA Filtration Media

- HEPA (High Efficiency Particulate Air) is a filtration standard developed by the US Atomic Energy Commission
- To be labelled a HEPA, a filter must remove dust and particulate matter ranging from 0.3 microns in size with 99.97% efficiency

Activated Carbon

- For VOC removal, activated carbon is like a sponge for gases
- Found either as a filter media impregnated with activated carbon or loose-fill granular carbon
- Granular activated carbons and other adsorbents are processed from either coconut shell, wood, coal, peat moss or zeolite

A combination of a HEPA filter and an activated carbon filter make the best type of filtration system. The HEPA will remove the dust, dander, pollens, molds, tobacco smoke etc., and the activated carbon will remove any VOCs and odours.

MANAGEMENT

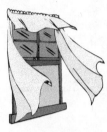

Improve Ventilation

Open a window, but remember the wind can carry troublesome particles. Air conditioning is an alternative. Air exchangers replace stale air with fresh; unfortunately they can also bring in undesirable contaminants from outside: pesticides, herbicides, air pollution and particularly woodsmoke. For very sensitive individuals, it is necessary to build in an additional charcoal filtration unit to eliminate pollutants. If you must work with questionable products (paint, etc.), do so in a well-ventilated area.

Before making any changes in your ventilation and filtration systems, consult a professional engineer familiar with the problem.

Create an Oasis

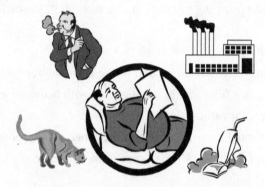

Like the oasis in a desert, at least one room in your home should provide a haven in harsh surroundings. Make this environment as free of problem items as possible (natural: dust, pollens, molds, and synthetic: SEA, formaldehyde, plastics). Spend time in this room just relaxing.

Establishing an oasis: begin with the bedroom and expand to include the entire house.

- Empty the room completely.
- Clean walls, floors, and windows with tolerated products.
- As you return articles to the room, question them for desirability. Does it smell? Has it been recently painted? Has it been treated with an insecticide?
- Use no floor covering, or use scatter rugs that can be washed frequently.
- Keep the bedroom closet free of dry-cleaned goods, toys, frequently worn shoes, sports equipment, and dirty clothing.
- Keep clutter, including magazines and newspapers, out.
- Clean the room regularly and thoroughly.
- Keep pets out.

If you are ill, you will feel better and if you are healthy, you're more likely to stay that way.

LET NATURE HELP YOU

PLANTS

Newly renovated homes, schools and offices emit many pollutants from new building materials as well as from new furniture. The Environmental Protection Agency (EPA) in the US found in a study that an 800 cu. ft. room (10 × 10 × 8) can generate a pollution level of 1.808 micrograms of formaldehyde, 112 micrograms of xylene, 67 micrograms of benzene. Dr. Bill C. Wolverton has studied plants at NASA for the past 25 years and found that certain plants have the ability to remove chemicals from indoor air. They absorb the toxins through their roots via soil minerals and leaves. On the following page is a table illustrating the toxin removal rate of some popular houseplants, adapted from an article written by Tina Spangler, in *Natural Health*.

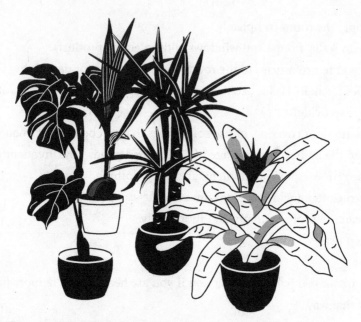

Toxin Removal Rate of Some Popular Houseplants

	FORMALDEHYDE	XYLENE	BENZENE	CARBON MONOXIDE
Boston Fern	1863 mcg/hr	208 mcg/hr		
English Ivy	1220 mcg/hr	131 mcg/hr	90% removed from a sealed chamber	
Areca Palm	938 mcg/hr	654 mcg/hr		
Spider Plant	560 mcg/hr	268 mcg/hr		96% removed from a sealed chamber
Striped Dracena	1361 mcg/hr	154 mcg/hr		

Attention: Plant soil can generate molds. Be sure to cover soil with one inch of activated charcoal. Do not use pesticides.

CHANGES IN LIFESTYLE

While these notes were written with the severely environmentally sensitive patient in mind, anyone can benefit.

1. Many individuals must change their lifestyle and start looking at all aspects of their life from a different perspective.
2. Go slowly, one step at a time. **Be realistic**; do only what you are able to.
3. Try staying with the rotation diet; a few slip-ups are human, but this diet is an important part of the treatment program. If you do slip up and have a reaction, this only confirms that foods are a problem.
4. Clean your house; create an oasis for you to come home to.
5. If you are planning to move, make sure you are not moving into a situation that is worse than the one you are in.
6. If you live in the city, take trips out to the countryside regularly to get away from pollution for a while.
7. A positive attitude does much to keep things in perspective, even on more difficult days.
8. Avoidance of offending substances, whenever possible, is the best advice for someone with sensitivities. Learn to say "no" when necessary.
9. Do not neglect your rest, nutrition and exercise.
10. If you are highly chemically sensitive, go shopping with a friend, who may see a reaction in you before you do.
11. Explore local sources of natural fibres, organic foods, and clean water.
12. Learn to read labels and to question manufacturers. Experiment with products to find out which ones you tolerate best.
13. Cooperate with your physician. Listen to what she says and question her if you are not sure of her explanation. You have to take an active role in your health. Remember: it's your body and you are responsible for it.
14. Support from friends and family is important for all of us. Share with them your efforts to regain your health. There are also several organizations promoting human ecology, which can provide you with practical information (See Resources).

MANAGEMENT

15. Work together, you do not need additional stress. If necessary, make an additional meeting with your doctor in order to explain your situation fully.

16. You will meet people, doctors included, who will raise their eyebrows and shake their heads: be prepared for this and be patient. However, you need not suffer abuse and ridicule. Find a doctor who understands the choices you want to make.

17. No one can actually know what you are going through, unless they have gone through it themselves.

18. Allergies never really disappear; they target another part of the body or bring about different symptoms, but they can be controlled or neutralized.

19. Remember that treatment and prevention are both essential. Being ecologically well includes a safe, clean environment, the rotation diet, desensitization, if necessary, exercise, awareness and a positive attitude. Remember that everyone is an individual; what works for one may not work for another, so you must search for viable alternatives for your own particular situation.

20. Keep in mind the overload phenomenon.

21. Never lose hope, instead keep busy, take things one step at a time and know your limits. Above all, do not be afraid to live; laughter is still the best medicine.

22. Always have faith in yourself and in a higher being. You *will* get better.

DETECTION OF PROBLEM ITEMS

To Detect a Problem in an Existing Room

Look again at the list of sources of formaldehydes, SEA and phenols, found on pages 97 to 106.

- Remove everything from the problem room and clean it.
- Replace items one at a time. As you do so, check for:

- exposed chipboard
- odours: mold, fragrance, tree terpens, formaldehyde
- synthetic fabrics and rubber
- dust collectors
- equipment in need of repair
- openings in walls and windows that may lead to mold
- At each stage of refitting, assess your comfort level
- Do not return problem items to the room

The Sniff Test

- If it smells good or bad, be cautious. Smell is one indication of outgassing. Pay attention to first impressions, as time goes on, we adjust to smell but not the effect.
- Heat the item slightly (smell is more obvious when warm), e.g., iron a shirt, run fabric under water, place an object in the sun. When you smell, be careful; waft the odour to your nose with a gentle hand motion.

The Challenge

- Remove yourself from the offending item for five to ten days. Watch for any reactions upon re-exposure.
- Place a sample of the questionable item into your oasis. Do you notice any difference in how you feel?

The Touch Test

- If a fabric feels harsh, uncomfortable or itchy, consider it a warning.

The Water Drop Test

- Generally the less treated a fabric, the more absorbent it will be.

The Mold Test

- Put slices of potato around the house. The speed of mold growth will tell you which rooms to clean first.

MANAGEMENT

TOWARDS AN ENVIRONMENTALLY SAFE HOME

Remember balance and moderation? One hundred percent safe is not possible. Do the best you can, setting goals that can be accomplished for short-term improvement, and then work towards long-term change, as you are able. The following pages outline points to be aware of in regards to various rooms. Highlight any points that apply to your home, and then make a plan of action.

Whatever the individual concerns might be, don't forget to establish a routine that will reduce dust, molds and chemicals that outgas.

General Considerations

- Consider wearing a mask when cleaning, as it will filter out the dust.
- Be aware of dust collectors (bookcases, dried and silk flowers, ornaments, decorative furnishings). Decrease the numbers and put items behind glass
- Wash drapes, pillows, bed covers, throw rugs.
- Clean behind and under furniture, not just around it.
- Control humidity.
- Low-odour latex paint is preferable to wallpaper or oil-based paint (unless you are allergic to latex).
- Decrease the number of plants (dust and mold collectors) and use activated carbon or crushed stone over the soil of those that remain.
- Wash all items (lamps, light bulbs, picture frames, fans).
- Install hardwood or ceramic floors and scatter rugs instead of wall-to-wall carpet. Wall to wall carpets can't be easily cleaned, they are often synthetic (petroleum based), treated with various chemicals (e.g., formaldehyde), prone to disintegration, and dust and dust mites accumulate underneath. They are unhygienic.
- Throw rugs should be free of chemical treatments and jute or rubber backing.
- Furnishings made of hardwood (oak, maple) or metal are best.

- Avoid sponge rubber and synthetic fabrics. Use cotton, kapok, or down to stuff furnishings.
- Gas and oil furnaces/appliances can cause problems. Replace oil furnaces with electric or high-efficiency gas models, but ensure adequate fresh air intake. Enclose the furnace in a room of its own. Clean ducts in all forced air heating systems a minimum of every three to five years.
- If you have forced air heating, keep the fan running continuously to prevent mold growth in ducts.
- Renovating: do some detective work first. Be sure your family tolerates the products used. Don't forget to ventilate the area and allow materials to gas off as much as possible before you spend any time in the room. Increasing the heat in the home for several days often speeds up the gassing off process.
- **Pest control: do not use pesticides or herbicides inside your home or on your lawn.**

Bedroom

- Most of us spend six to eight hours in this room each day; make it a top priority for your clean up. Take the time to create an oasis and you will be amazed at what a trouble free sleep can do for you. Think of this room as a place to sleep and relax; keep items unrelated to these activities somewhere else.
- Use natural, untreated fibres (cotton, linen, wool, silk) for bedding, drapes, rug and other linens. Wash regularly.
- Replace polyester and foam pillows with organic cotton or organic buckwheat pillows, kapok or even cotton towels. If dust mites are a problem, then use dust-mite proof pillow casings.
- Keep toys (particularly plush or stuffed), knick-knacks, books, and dust collectors to a minimum.
- For easy cleaning, space under the bed should be free of boxes and stored articles.

- If you have pets or plants, keep them out of this room.
- Put a barrier sheet cover over your mattress to keep out dust and mites. Use cotton, not vinyl. There are special anti-mite covers. Remember to test for tolerance.
- When shopping for a new washer, consider the European type, which heats the water to a boiling temperature that kills the dust mites.
- Avoid foam mattresses and waterbeds.* Both are prime mold growth areas and can also be problems for the chemically sensitive. Try a metal box spring and cotton mattress instead. For a short-term measure, use cotton sheets to create a natural barrier between yourself and the mattress.
- Avoid plywood and chipboard furnishings or seal unlaminated sides with Crystal Shield or other safe water-based urethane if tolerable.
- Keep dirty laundry in another room, as perspiration favours mold growth and fabrics often attract chemical odours (e.g., perfume).
- Avoid using your bedroom closet as a storage cupboard. Use a cotton garment bag instead of a vinyl one.
- Minimize the amount of dry-cleaning you do and do not keep dry cleaned items in your bedroom, as the solvents used are toxic; better yet, find a "green clean" cleaner.
- Avoid electric blankets.*
  * water beds and electric blankets are a major source of electromagnetic radiation and can be hazardous.

Bathroom

- Clean tiles, grouting, caulking, shower curtain, floor by the toilet bowl base, and the toilet tank. Zephrin and Borax both help discourage mold growth.
- Use a fabric shower curtain instead of a plastic one. Be aware that shower doors are prone to mold growth.
- Dry down the shower stall after use.

- Good ventilation is important; a fan, a window that opens.
- Use cotton towels and washcloths. Dry out towels and bath mats.
- Avoid coloured/perfumed tissues.
- Use and store only tolerated personal care products. Be wary of odourous products (e.g., soaps, deodorants, powders, hairspray, shaving foam, nail polish, cosmetics, perfumes). Even with the lid on, many of these gas off.

Laundry

- Use only tolerated cleaning products (e.g., Borax, Nature Clean Laundry Detergent, or other unscented product)
- Be sure this area is well ventilated.

Closets

- Air contents regularly.
- Install a fan or light to reduce mold growth in prone areas.

Basement/Garage

When attached to the home, the garage must be treated like any other room. Fumes from cars, activities and stored items seep into the house via walls, doors, and the ceiling. The same thing applies to the basement. For this reason be very aware of what and how you store items. If possible, the items listed below should be kept elsewhere.

- garden products, rubber hoses, sprays, lawn mower
- car parts, oil, antifreeze
- books, magazines, old clothing, furniture and other unused items
- paints, thinners, shellacs, glues, scrap lumber (chip board, plywood), styrofoam
- consider letting the car cool down outside before moving it into the garage

MANAGEMENT

If the area is damp: use a dehumidifier, improve cross-ventilation. Repair cracks in walls and floor and use effective storage methods. **Prevent flooding of the basement. If it does happen, clean completely, remove the carpet and allow to dry thoroughly.**

Kitchen

- Use electric appliances rather than gas.
- Watch for molds: plants, cold water pipes, molding around sink, dry rack tray, refrigerator, and cupboards under the sink.
- Use a marble block or wooden chopping board that can be washed in hot soapy water.
- Clean with Borax.
- Improve ventilation.
- If the area under the sink is prone to moisture, minimize use of this area.
- Bare floor, no rugs.
- Keep garbages clean.
- Remove odourous and otherwise offensive cleaning products (fabric softeners, oven cleaners, floor wax, polishes).
- Keep the refrigerator free of leftovers and spoiled foods. Clean all parts regularly.
- Avoid plastics. The plasticizers used in their production tend to leach into foods and liquids stored within. (e.g., plastic containers, plastic wrap). If you must use them, hard plastics are better tolerated than soft.
- Use stainless steel or Corning Ware for cooking. **Avoid aluminum** as studies have shown that it is toxic when heated and aluminum has been linked to Alzheimer's disease.

MICROWAVE OVENS

These appliances emit low energy radiation as do TVs and computers. Some research indicates the harmful effects of low-level electromagnetic radiation. Many patients who are chemically and food sensitive have reported that they can tolerate foods cooked by microwave better than using other appliances. It has to be remembered, however, that microwave ovens change the molecular structure of food and deplete nutrients.

Your Work Environment

Many individuals spend a sizeable chunk of their time on the job. In order to do our best, we need to be able to think clearly, concentrate, and feel well enough to perform our daily duties. The environment (physical and psychological) we work in has a great deal to do with how we feel. A traumatic day at work can leave you feeling tired and irritable and can contribute markedly to your total body load. Add to this an energy-efficient work area with no fresh air and pollutants from photocopiers, synthetic furnishings, cleaning products, dust, mold, bacteria, perfume, and tobacco smoke. **The end result: ill employees, excessive sick leaves, poor mental performance, mistakes, loss of productivity, and ultimately loss of income. For the environmentally sensitive, any work place involves challenges that need be addressed.**

If you work at home, you have control over the offending items and can make your work environment as safe as your leisure rooms. For the majority of us, changes at work may be more difficult to achieve; however, even small modifications can make a difference. Also worth remembering is the fact that a "safe" home is a haven to return to at the end of the day. It can serve to balance some of the stresses you encounter at work.

Improving Your Office

- Help individuals become more aware. Talk to your supervisor; write a letter to management, present a letter from your doctor if you think it might help.
- Keep a written record of any communication you receive regarding air quality.
- Circulate a petition to bring the matter to the attention of officials. Keep it positive; remember a healthier workplace means more productive employees.

MANAGEMENT

- Talk to your union.
- **If you are the manager, initiate changes that will benefit everyone.**
- During renovations or use of pesticides, you have the right to stay off work; check with your local office of the Ministry of Labour.
- If your needs cannot be accommodated and you are getting more symptoms, a change of workplace is recommended.
- Take a walk at lunch or break time. Some stretching, light exercise, and fresh air will increase your energy level.
- Use a humidifier to help fight dry air, and drink tolerated water throughout the day.
- Keep your office environment clean.
- Consider spider plants; they actually absorb formaldehyde.
- Use a portable air cleaner. A small fan might also help remove stale air.
- Move your desk away from odourous machines (e.g., photocopiers).
- Talk to your co-workers about your sensitivity to perfume and tobacco smoke, but don't harp on it. Keep the tone positive.
- Keep your desk clean. Clear the top each night to discourage a build-up of paper and dust.
- Use safe products, e.g., water-based markers, white glue.
- A private office may eliminate some environmental offenders, and you can successfully use a portable air filter.
- Bring your lunch to avoid cafeteria lunch.

Don't give up! As the saying goes, *"slow and steady wins the race."* However, remember that trying to convince maintenance management to make changes is often very difficult, and getting compensation for loss of work due to environmental sensitivities is almost impossible.

A SPECIAL NOTE ON COMPUTERS

Computers are now widely used, but research into the health effects of working with them are still in their infancy. Three concerns have been expressed:

1. Physical arrangement of work stations is important from two perspectives; computer glare leading to eye problems, and posture, creating musculoskeletal pains.
2. Electromagnetic radiation is emitted from the computer monitors. Some individuals are concerned about exposure to the user. Newer models, built according to stricter international standards, emit less radiation.
3. Low frequency waves (electromagnetic) can be emitted from the sides or the backs of other computers around you.

Problems that may be associated with monitors:

- eye strain, burning eyes, blurred vision, headaches
- stomach upset and nausea
- back, neck and shoulder pain; repetitive strain disorder
- CNS and endocrine disturbances (pineal gland— circadian rhythms)

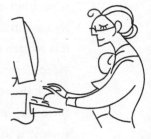

Safe practices when using a computer include:

- Using new as opposed to old equipment.
- Using a well-ventilated, uncarpeted room (computers outgas and carpets cause static).
- Extremely sensitive persons could use an exhaust hood over the unit.
- Using an air purifier.
- Good lighting (less than is necessary for reading a book).
- No glare.
- Proper glasses (glasses set to the distance of the monitor are better than bifocals).
- An ergonomically designed chair that helps maintain good posture.
- Taking breaks and exercising (at least a 15-minute break every 2 hours).
- Alternate between computer work and other work.
- Move the keyboard 2 to 3 feet from the screen.

MANAGEMENT

- Place the monitor in a metal cabinet or surround it with wire mesh to create an electric shield.

THE SCHOOL ENVIRONMENT

Just as adults can be aggravated by their work environment, children can experience symptoms due to factors within the classroom or school. The following are some thoughts that might prove helpful in dealing with your child's school, particularly if your child is highly sensitive.

- Share information with your child's teacher, the principal, and the school nurse. Dr. Doris Rapp's book entitled *The Impossible Child* is a well-summarized account of allergies as they relate to children, and it is written for parents and teachers alike. Rapp has also produced a video, *Environmentally Sick Schools*, which can be used as a resource. Check the school environment for possible hazards. Remember that there is a fine line between being overprotective and not being aware of situations that cause reactions.

- Help your children to understand their sensitivities, but don't make them feel unusual; rather teach them to understand their limits.

- If your child cannot participate in a planned activity, have an alternative available.

- Have the child bring all foods from home. If an event or party requires a snack, try sending one that other children might also enjoy. (A prescription of Nalcrom [sodium cromoglycate] may help the child tolerate sensitive foods on special occasions.) **This does not apply to food allergies that cause anaphylaxis. These foods should *never* be eaten.**

- Place the child's desk away from an air vent, preferably near a window. Also try to keep the child's desk at a distance from the chalkboard.

- Encourage the child to tell his/her teacher if feeling unwell.

- If the child cannot go out for recess, provide him/her with some other meaningful activity.

MANAGEMENT

- Encourage the use of alternatives to toxic paints, glues and magic markers, and establish safe practices with all art materials.
- Any medications that must be administered throughout the day should be left at the school, along with explicit directions regarding its administration.
- If a child is having a reaction, the assisting adult must remain calm. It will further upset the child if he/she sees that the adult is upset.
- Children (and adults) who have severe reactions to substances should wear a medical identification bracelet.
- It is wise to let the teacher or whoever is in charge know what type of reaction your child might have and any early signals. This may help avert a reaction before it becomes severe. **If your child has anaphylactic reactions, make sure the teachers know how to administer an Epipen, which the child or school should have available at all times.**
- It may be advisable to get the co-operation of the staff, classmates and their parents to keep anaphylaxis-causing foods out of your child's classroom, and possibly the whole school.
- **There is no excuse for any individual school to start renovation or painting during the academic year. Two months' summer vacation is sufficient to get the work done. You may request postponement of any such work from your school for medical reasons.**
- There is also no excuse for use of toxic chemicals for maintenance. Use of pesticides in and around the school should be prohibited. These chemicals are very potent, and their effect on growing organisms is particularly dangerous. Educate your school and school board.
- If ventilation is at fault, attempts should be made to correct the problems, and use of portable air filters should be instituted in the meantime.
- There are boards in Ontario, particularly in the Kitchener-Waterloo area, which recognize the problem of indoor air pollution in schools and have created environmentally safe classrooms for children who suffer from environmental hypersensitivity disorders. Of course, **all classrooms in all schools should be environmentally safe for all**

MANAGEMENT

students and all teachers. Physical health, behaviour and cognitive learning would improve all around.

- If your child is housed in a portable classroom, inspect it yourself and ask for documentation that shows that it has been inspected and cleared of any mold. Even if your child is not experiencing symptoms, if mold is present, it may contribute to detrimental health effects down the road.

ALTERNATIVE PERSONAL CARE PRODUCTS

Many personal care and household products contain synthetic chemicals that are troublesome for the environmentally sensitive person. Fortunately, safer alternatives are available. Shop in natural food stores and holistic pharmacies for fragrance-free, hypoallergenic products. Listed below are some of the common offenders and options many patients can tolerate. Be sure to read the labels.

Please note:

- in some cases, avoidance is the safest measure
- each individual must consider his/her own tolerance; no product is 100% safe for everyone
- natural products can have strong odours, e.g., peppermint, lavender, etc.

Where To Purchase Environmentally Safe Products

- Health food stores
- Alternative sections of grocery stores
- Healthy Home Services Inc.—unique collection of products personally selected and tested from a variety of manufacturers equally concerned about negative health and ecosystem effects from chronic exposure to chemicals often found in conventional products. Tel: 613-623-0933 or 1-800-819-1598.
- Consult *the Safe Shopper's Bible: a Consumer's Guide to Nontoxic House-hold Products, Cosmetics and Food*. David Steinman & Samuel S. Epstein, MD. MacMillan 1995.

MANAGEMENT

Perfumes and Perfumed Products (see also p. 125)

Perfume, Cologne, Astringent	· Do not use these products at all, or at least rarely, and even then with great subtlety
Hair Shampoo, Conditioner	· Choose a shampoo with very little or no odour or perfume Remember some herbal shampoos still have odour, see if you tolerate it
Deodorant, Antiperspirant	· Choose a deodorant without scent and aluminum · Baking soda (aluminum-free) can always be used · Rock mineral crystals are available, along with other scent-free products
Soap	· Look for a soap that is perfume-free, such as pure glycerin soap
Hair Spray	· Use a hairstyle that requires no spray · Look for unscented gels or mousse
Cosmetics	· look for fragrance-free, hypoallergenic products
Shaving Cream, Aftershave	· look for fragrance-free, hypoallergenic products
Lotions	· look for fragrance-free, hypoallergenic products Choose one that you tolerate.
Mosquito Repellant	· Citronella, vitamin B_1
Sunscreen	· Try to cover up with hats and clothing as much as possible · Titanium dioxide and zinc applied to the skin provide an effective block · If necessary, use a commercial sunscreen that works effectively with the least amount of chemicals · Supplement with Vitamins A, C, D and E.

MANAGEMENT

Alternative Household Cleaning Products

PRODUCTS	ALTERNATIVES
Laundry Detergents	• e.g., Nature Clean Laundry Powder or Liquid • Nature Clean Laundry Bleach Powder–a 100% chlorine-free laundry bleach, or their Liquid Non-chlorine Bleach (hydrogen peroxide and water) • Washing or baking Soda • Other unscented laundry products
Fabric Softeners for Natural Fibres	• 1 cup of vinegar or $\frac{1}{4}$ cup baking soda added to the final rinse • e.g., Nature Clean Natural Fabric Softener
Fabric Stain Removers	• End-it (bar) • e.g., Nature Clean Laundry Stain Remover • Hydrogen peroxide based bleach replacements also remove stains
Disinfectants: e.g., Lysol, Pinesol	• e.g., Zephrin (1:750 solution); ask for it at your pharmacy. Concentrate is also available. • e.g., Nature Clean Non-chlorine Bleach–makes a great general purpose disinfectant. • e.g., Hydrox 2: Hydrogen Peroxide Based Cleaner–user friendly / low emission (available from Virox–1-800-387-7578, www.virox.com) • OxiClean, a hydrogen peroxide and oxygen cleaner–www.greatcleaners.com
Abrasive Cleaners: e.g., Spic & Span Scrub & Shine Comet, Ajax	• Sodium bicarbonate (baking soda) • Washing soda (Arm & Hammer) • Shaklee products (Basic I and Basic H) are odour-free concentrated cleaners • Tri-sodium phosphate
Floor and Furniture Polish/Wax	• Olive oil: lemon juice (2:1) • Water spots–10 drops lemon oil in 2 cups vodka, rub into spot and dry immediately
Oven Cleaners	• Washing soda, water and steel wool • e.g., Nature Clean Oven & Barbecue Cleaner

MANAGEMENT

PRODUCTS	ALTERNATIVES
Room Deodorizers, Air Fresheners	• Air filters, baking soda • Zeolite (an abundant, natural volcanic rock that is 100% non-toxic to people and pets. Its unique crystal structure makes it highly efficient at eliminating odours.
Silver Cleaner	• Dissolve 1 tbsp. baking soda in 1 quart of near boiling water, place silver in aluminum pan or pan with aluminum foil. Be sure all pieces are immersed in the solution. Let sit several minutes, then rinse and dry.
Upholstery Cleaners	• Zephiran liquid • Water and vinegar • e.g., Nature Clean Carpet & Upholstery Cleaner—a unique hypoallergenic alternative to the solvent formulas

Alternatives for Other Household Products

PRODUCTS	ALTERNATIVES
Moth Balls	• If you can tolerate tree terpenes, use a cedar chest for linens. Cedar eggs also help. • Cloves have been reported as effective • Store clean items only and air in the sun or run through a warm dryer periodically • Washing destroys all forms of the moth
Bug Sprays	• Prevent problems by keeping home clean and free of items attractive to pests, e.g., food crumbs, clutter • Use adhesive pest traps, thereby avoiding aerosols
Glues and Adhesives	• White glue—all purpose • School glue—Borden's Elmer's
Pens, Markers, Inks	• Use water-based inks and markers, non-scented
Liquid Paper	• Use corrections tape instead
Dry Cleaning Fluids	• Minimize use, air out thoroughly before wearing any clothes treated in this way • Find an environmentally safe cleaner that uses water instead of chemical solvents • Federal government may be phasing out dry cleaning completely

MANAGEMENT

PRODUCTS	ALTERNATIVES
Synthetic Clothing	• Many have a strong formaldehyde odour, particularly when new or heated. Wash before wearing. • Choose natural untreated fibres such as cotton, linen, wool, and silk • Organic cotton is now available in a wide variety of applications from bedding to personal clothing
Paints	• Latex is preferable to oil-based paint, however, refer back to page 128 if you have a latex allergy. • All painting is best done when the area can be aired thoroughly, and, if possible, allow it to gas off for at least two weeks before moving back into the environment. • Benjamin Moore, C.I.L., Glidden produce low-odour paints • Choose pastel colours to keep the odour low
Stains	• Quite often have extreme odour, but can be sealed afterwards. Water-based always preferable.
Finishes	• Crystal Shield (floor finish) and Crystal Aire (furniture finish) http://www.nontoxic.com Tel: 1 800 968 9355 or http://poloplaz.com Tel: 1-800421-7319 • Choose a water-based product, and it will have far less odour during the application and afterwards

MANAGEMENT

WATER

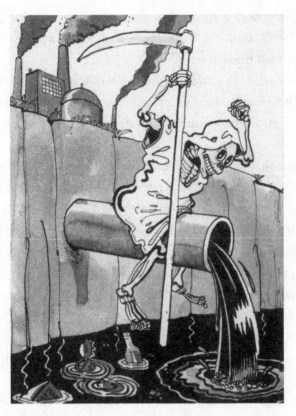

Artist: Andrzej Mleczko
From: Ecologia (or how to love nature), Krakow, Poland 1991

Facts

- Water comprises two thirds of our body weight. It assists with the transportation of nutrients and other substances throughout the body.
- We require a constant supply of fresh water, or dehydration will result. It is suggested that we drink at least eight glasses of water per day.
- Not only do we drink water, but also we ingest it in our foods (watermelon, for instance, is 95% water).
- We also absorb water through our skin (e.g., in the shower).
- "Hard" water contains calcium and magnesium. The mineral content makes it a good drinking water, and it helps to prevent atherosclerosis.

The Water Question...Is It Safe?

- A large percentage of the world's water comes from underground sources (wells, aquifers). Some also comes from surface water, such as lakes and man-made reservoirs.

- Environmental toxins affect both sources of water, adding unwanted chemicals to our precious water supply. In addition, chlorine and fluoride are often added to municipal water, causing a problem for some individuals.

- Fluoride should not be in water at all, and the danger with the addition of chlorine to water is the resultant by-products that it produces. Chlorine reacts with natural, organic material (e.g., decaying leaves) present in untreated water to form THMs (Trihalomethanes) and other chlorinated by-products. The most common THMs found in drinking water are chloroform, bromodichloromethane, chlorodibromomethane and bromoform. These by-products are a concern to us because human population studies have shown that chlorinated drinking water, high in THM levels, may be associated with a slight increase in certain types of cancer following long-term exposure (more than 35 years.*)

  * *THMs in Our Drinking Water, Nov. 1995 from Ministry of Environment and Energy, Fax-on-Demand Publications.*

There are five key groups of toxic substances that can cause contamination:
1. Particulates (e.g., sand, rust)
2. Dissolved Inorganics (e.g., heavy metals, asbestos)
3. Organics (e.g., chemical solvents, PCBs)
4. Radiological contaminants
5. Biological pathogens (e.g., viruses bacteria, parasites),

As stated in the section dealing with chemicals, one thousand chemicals have been identified in the Great Lakes. In Lake Ontario alone, there are over 250 toxic chemicals.

MANAGEMENT

In addition, forty percent of Ontario wells are contaminated with pesticides and herbicides.

As a result of the questionable quality of our tap water more and more people are searching for alternatives. However, the manufacture and sale of water treatment devices for home use are unregulated in Canada. And, unfortunately, so is the sale of bottled water.

Water Treatment Alternatives

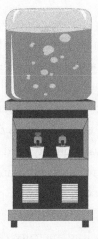

I look good, and smell good,   *but am I safe?*

There are both positive and negative aspects to each option. In the end, individuals must find a drinking water that they can tolerate.

Bottled Water

- natural mineral content is retained
- the source of the spring must be questioned
- plastic contaminates the water stored in it
- avoid soft plastic containers for your water

Reverse Osmosis

Reverse osmosis is a multi-stage treatment system involving mechanical filtration, activated carbon absorption, and reverse osmosis. The units are

MANAGEMENT

designed to force pressurized water through a microscopic membrane, which rejects contaminants suspended in the water. This membrane permits passage of the improved water to a holding tank. A consequence of this technique is that a lot of water is wasted, adding to its cost. Reverse osmosis is excellent for removal of dirt, toxic metals, fluorides, nitrates and sodium, asbestos, pesticides and herbicides, chlorine, THMs, bacteria and microorganisms. However, it will also remove minerals (e.g., calcium, copper, chromium, selenium, zinc, etc.) from the water.

Activated Carbon Filter

Activated carbon filters are more effective in the solid form rather than the loose granular form. The surface of a molecule of carbon electrically attracts and holds on to chemical molecules. The solid forms have a much larger surface area than the loose forms and can therefore absorb and hold on to more water contaminants. Regular changes of the cartridge (every 7 to 8 months depending on your water quality) and internal cleaning/disinfecting of the cartridge housing assure consistent water quality.

Solid carbon block filters will remove suspended solids (e.g., sand, silt, sediment, rust etc.) down to 0.5 microns in size. Chlorine, THMs, volatile organic chemicals, pesticides, lead, mercury, cadmium, certain bacteria and parasites will also be removed, leaving behind minerals. However, this does not remove flouride.

Distillation

Water is boiled; the steam is then cooled, condensed and collected. Toxic organic and volatile gases with a boiling point lower than water re-contaminate the distilled water. Fractional distillers try to prevent this by venting volatile gases prior to condensation.

A vented distiller will remove chemicals, heavy metals, nitrates, fluoride, chlorine and its by-products, rust and sediment, but will also remove all minerals.

Ultraviolet Water Sterilizer

Ultraviolet light applications are generally used as an adjunct for under-sink and reverse osmosis point-of-use filtration systems. Disinfection is achieved by exposing filtered water to germicidal ultraviolet light at a normal water flow rate. Short wave UV light (256 nanometers) destroys bacteria, viruses and other microorganisms by interfering with DNA and RNA in the organism's reproduction cycle.

Choosing the Right System

Many models exist today; check your phone book, under Water Purification Equipment, for the retailers near you. Everything from portable sink units and permanent units, to whole home filtration systems are available. Keep in mind that your skin is also an absorption site for chemicals, so improvements with showering or bathing can be made with whole home or shower filters. Remember, no two people are alike. You must find the system that best suits YOUR needs. Remember also that it is a totally unregulated business and it's always a good idea to get a second opinion.

Controlling Humidity

Anyone who has experienced a hot day in August knows how uncomfortable this can be, but did you know that these conditions are ideal breeding grounds for mold? On the other hand, too little moisture in the air also leads to difficulties, particularly during the winter, when house dust levels rise and particles cling to electrostatically charged surfaces.

Ideal relative humidity levels for a home are in the range of 40% to 60%.

A dry environment can be fixed at the source by improving vapour barriers, insulation, and weather-stripping as these measures will decrease heating requirements and conserve moisture in the air. If these measures do not produce effective results, a humidifier may be required. Many types of humidifiers can be found on the market. Steer clear of models that work by evaporation, as they are ideal breeding grounds. If you use an ultrasonic

MANAGEMENT

model, be sure to add only distilled or filtered water to prevent spraying toxic chemicals into the air you breathe.

If excess humidity is the problem, increased airflow and good ventilation are the best solution, although dehumidifiers are helpful.

Note: Humidifiers and dehumidifiers are ideal breeding grounds for molds and viruses; clean them daily! Membrane-type or drum-type humidifiers in your furnaces are unacceptable. Use a jet-type humidifier.

Air Filters

As with water filters, many varieties of air filters are available, in varying sizes and at different prices. As discussed earlier, HEPA (High Efficiency Particulate Air Cleaners) filters are the most efficient in removal of dust and particulate matter down to 0.3 microns. When coupled with an activated carbon filter, it will also address odours and volatile organic compounds. A good quality HEPA filter may restrict air flow on a furnace and damage the motor, but you will find free standing units, powered with their own heavy duty motor, that are very efficient.

Individual sensitivities must also be taken into consideration and for some, testing of the different types of carbon used in the units may be necessary. For the allergic person it is recommended that a portable air cleaner be capable of changing the air in a room (preferably the bedroom) six to eight times per hour. A metal housing is a must, as plastics or vinyl will off-gas VOCs.

Some brand names that display these qualities are ALLERAIR, AUSTIN AIR HEALTHMATE, and AMAIRCARE, to name a few. Car travel can be very difficult for some environmentally sensitive people. Consider a car air cleaner to ease travelling. Portable units can be purchased that plug into the cigarette lighter, and most come with an adapter that allows them to be used in hotel rooms, for example.

MANAGEMENT

TRAVEL TIPS FOR THE SENSITIVE INDIVIDUAL

Car Travel

1. Air conditioning in a car is helpful; buy the type with a recirculating air feature in order to prevent pulling in road and engine fumes through the vents. Some models (e.g., BMW, Ford, GM and some Japanese makes) filter the air through charcoal during the recirculation of the air. However, also be aware that certain molds (such as cladosporium, penicillium, aureobasidium, aspergillus, etc.) can colonize air conditioning or evaporator units in cars. Have your air conditioning unit checked in your car if you are arriving unwell to your destination.

2. Open all the windows and doors to let the car air out as long as possible before starting the motor.

3. Close the windows, start the motor, and begin to drive before turning on the air-conditioner.

4. After the car is in motion, drive with the windows open and the air-conditioning set on high for five or ten minutes to allow any mold that has gathered in the air conditioner overnight to be dispersed by the wind.

5. Close all the windows again and keep your air conditioner on maximum cool if caught in traffic or heavy pollution.

6. Keep the air filter clean.

7. Take as many back roads as possible to avoid heavy pollution.

8. Plug in a portable air purifier to help absorb off-gassing vapours as well as exhaust fumes.

9. Do not use the heater except when absolutely necessary.

10. If sensitive to a soft vinyl interior, cover the seats with old cotton mattress pads and untreated cotton. This will help keep down the fumes released by heat, sun and the human body. Denim and sailcloth make good covers.

MANAGEMENT

11. Start your trip early in the morning. If travelling from a populated area, plan to leave when the traffic is light.

12. Happily, most airlines now have smoke-free flights. If travelling by air, choose a non-smoking flight or at least be sure to obtain a non-smoking seat. If oxygen is necessary, make all the arrangements well ahead of time. Be sure to mention that a ceramic mask is to be used. A doctor's note may be necessary.

13. Always travel with some of your own tolerated food and water, and look into the possibility of airlines providing special meal preparation.

Hotels and Motels

Nothing will spoil a trip or holiday faster than becoming sick due to unhealthy accommodations. One night is all it takes to bring on the sore throats and flu-like symptoms.

Listed below are some simple precautions to use when arranging accommodation:

1. Pick your hotel wisely. Learn to read brochures from a new perspective. "Newly renovated" should translate as "avoid." Tile floors are preferable to "plush carpeting." Make sure windows can open. A balcony is nice. Bring your own linens if you are particularly sensitive to commercial detergents or synthetic bedding.

2. Call the hotel ahead of time and find out what kind of arrangements they can help you make, e.g., kitchenettes, non-smoking and non-carpeted rooms,

3. The higher the ceiling, the better the air.

4. Request a room that has not been fumigated recently and has no air fresheners. Ask staff to open a window and air the room before you get there.

5. Pick accommodation off the highway or main thoroughfare, as there will likely be less pollution.

6. Take along any personal safe products or articles that may be difficult to find on the road.

7. Carry Zephrin with you to wash down walls etc. in the washroom in case of mold.

8. Bring your own portable room air cleaner.

IF YOU MUST USE PESTICIDES...

Obviously you are urged not to use pesticides at all—for your own health, the health of your families and the health of this earth and all creatures therein. However, if for some reason you really must do so, at least take these precautions:

- Read the label before buying or using pesticides; use pesticides only for purposes listed and in the manner directed.
- Do not apply more than the specified amount of pesticide. Overdoses can harm you and the environment.
- Keep pesticides away from food and dishes.
- Keep children and pets away from pesticides and sprayed areas.
- Avoid inhalation of pesticides.
- Do not spray outdoors on a windy day.
- If a pesticide is spilled on clothing, wash with soap and water and change clothing immediately.
- If a pesticide is swallowed, check the label for first-aid treatment. Call or go to the doctor or hospital immediately, keeping the pesticide label with you.

PEST CONTROL WITHOUT PESTICIDES...

Here are some hints to control ants, cockroaches, flies and termites. First things first: cleanliness is still next to godliness, don't leave any crumbs or garbage around which can attract them.

MANAGEMENT

Ants

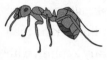

- Pour boiling water on the colony of ants
- Ant drops (liquid ant killer containing Borax)
- Diatomaceous earth
- Wipe up a line of ants with a wet sponge so that other ants will not follow
- Sprinkle powdered chili pepper, paprika, dried peppermint or borax where ants enter
- Plant mint around the outside of the house to discourage ants from entering.

Cockroaches

- Mix equal parts baking soda, boric acid and powdered sugar. Spread lightly around infested area. This will kill roaches.
- Use cucumber rinds or bay leaves in infested area. This will repel roaches.
- Use diatomaceous earth (e.g., Fossil Flower®)
- Use roach motel
- Chinese chalk

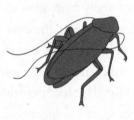

Flies

- Use screens on windows and doors.
- Buy sticky flypaper made of a mixture of boiled sugar, corn syrup and water on brown paper. This can even be made at home.
- Hang clusters of cloves in a room if fragrance tolerated. This repels flies.
- Citrus oil released from scraped orange will repel flies.

Spider mites

- Place fresh banana peels in infested areas. Fresh banana peel contains a volatile aldehyde that is toxic to spider mites. To sustain the effect, replace with fresh banana peel regularly.

MANAGEMENT

- Spray 10% butyl alcohol and water onto infested areas. This is an effective mitocide, which lasts for three to six months.

Termites:
- Use heat. Apply 140 degrees for 10 minutes with a heat lamp.

Fleas:
- Feed your pet brewer's yeast with food. The B vitamins create an odour fleas abhor.
- Diatomaceous earth is a safe flea killer, sprinkled on fur or on floors.
- When bathing pets, ensure fleas go down the drain.

Resource: The Bug Busters, *by Bernice Lifton, Avery Publishing Group, 1991.*
TheCookbook Decoder, *by Arthur Grosser,78 rpm Press, 1988.*

NATURAL PEST CONTROL PRODUCTS

With growing awareness about the harm toxic pesticides and herbicides do to the earth and our health, in addition to time-tested home remedies, there are now many products available to help you safely in your home and garden. These include herbal remedies, natural insect traps and lures, repellants, beneficial insects, etc. Most garden centers now carry many natural or at least less toxic products such as insecticidal soaps and biological pesticides, which have fewer harmful side effects but are still poisons and should be used with care and not as a first choice.

Read your labels carefully. For example, the following terms may be confusing. **Pyrethrum** refers to a powder made from the dried flowers of the Chrysanthemum plant. **Pyrethrin** refers to six different insecticide compounds that occur naturally in the Pyrethrum powder. While natural, these are nonetheless powerful insecticides, can cause allergic reactions and are toxic to aquatic life. **Permethrin** refers to the synthetically produced version of Pyrethrum, and the term **Perethroids** refers to the synthetic equivalent of the six natural Pyrethrins. They are neurotoxic, carcinogenic, hormone-disrupting and highly toxic to aquatic life and bees.

MANAGEMENT

SPECIAL NOTE ON HEAD LICE:

Permethrin (see above), Lindane (a chlorinated hydrocarbon poison banned in 18 countries) and Malathion (an organophosphate) are carcignogenic and neurotoxic and are common ingredients in anti-lice products available over the counter or by prescription. Lice are becoming resistant to them. Children, however, are *not* resistant to these poisons! *Please* find and use the following alternatives for your children: *Follicel*, a non-toxic hypoallergenic product used in Europe for years and now available in North American (**www.bibiheadlice.com**), *Treemenda Tea Tree Oil* products (**www.treemenda .com**), *Not Nice to Lice* (**www.notnice2lice.com**).

In addition to information from your local health food store or naturally-inclined garden center, following are some numbers and websites where information and/or catalogues are available:

- Integrated BioSystems Inc., 1-877-501-5003 **www.integratedbiosys.com**
- Kanata Environmental Network based in Ottawa
  www.kanataenvironmentalnetwork.com
- Planet Natural, 1-800-289-6656 **www.planetnatural.com**
- Safe 2 Use – (909) 372-9850 **www.safe2use.com**
- Vermont Country Store, 1-800-931-9916 ext. 100
  www.vermontcountrystore.com
- Victor Poison Free®, Safer®, Havahart® products: 1-800-800-1819
  www.victorpest.com with link to Woodstream Canada site:
  www.victorpest.com/canada

ORGANIC LAWN CARE

You can have a healthy, lush lawn without the use of chemical pesticides. Here are some lawn care tips that are recommended by Toronto Environmental Alliance and Greenpeace:

Steps to Organic Lawn Care

1. **Aerate:** if your soil is compacted, aerate in the spring and/or fall before fertilizing and seeding to increase air and water circulation.

2. **Topdress:** after aerating and weeding and before seeding, spread top-soil and/or composted manure/finished compost over your entire lawn. This adds nutrients and microorganisms to your lawn.

3. **Overseed:** overseed every year in spring or late summer during cool moist conditions to replace dying grass plants.

4. **Mow:** research at the University of Guelph demonstrated that 3 inches is an ideal height for turf grass because it shades out weeds, which prefer more sunny and open locations, and also shades the soil, keeping it cool and moist.

5. **Water:** water deeply (about 1 inch) in the early morning or early evening once a week to encourage deep roots.

6. **Mulch:** use grass clippings as a perfect fertilizer for lawns; they can boost soil fertility by up to 30 percent.

7. **Monitor:** monitor your lawn for insects, weeds and diseases. If a problem develops, take necessary "natural" action.

8. **Rake:** raking increases air circulation and discourages fungal growth. Rake after grass dries out, but before weed seeds start to germinate in earnest.

9. **Fertilize:** fertilize naturally, such as finished compost, grass clippings and/or slow-release organic products (e.g., well-aged manure and seaweed). Organic fertilizers are best applied in late summer/early fall, but may also be used in the early spring. Compost and grass clippings can be applied throughout the growing season.

10. **Novel Idea:** Plant flowers/herbs/trees/ground cover and vegetables instead of grass. *A monoculture lawn is an unnatural ecosystem.*

FOUR-DAY ROTARY DIVERSIFIED DIET

In a previous chapter, the topic of food sensitivity/allergy was discussed. In this section of the book, we will look at how to control the problem. The most obvious solution would be to avoid a troublesome food, thus avoiding the reactions caused by it. This is effective for recognized sensitivities. In fact, it is recommended that packaged, processed, convenience foods also be avoided as they often contain hidden food ingredients (wheat, milk, eggs, corn, sugar, etc.). Above all, avoid the four "W"s: white bread, white flour, white sugar, white rice. Unfortunately, avoidance alone is usually not enough. Why? Remember the concept of cyclical food sensitivities: overexposure to any one food leads to the development of a problem with that food. For the environmentally sensitive, this is a definite possibility unless efforts are made to introduce more variety into the diet. The key to food allergy management is the "rotary diversified diet," as it helps to prevent food sensitivities. Please note that in some cases your doctor may recommend neutralization therapy for key foods, or use EPD treatment.

Basic Principles of the Rotary Diversified Diet:

Individual foods, together with their biological families, are rotated following a four-day cycle.

Let's look at an example: Jane is following a rotation diet. For breakfast on Monday, she decided to have scrambled eggs. That day at lunch, she had cold chicken and then chicken soup for dinner. For the next three days, she will avoid chicken, eggs, and all related foods, and on day five, Jane will choose from these items again. To keep things simple, rather than keeping track of when she last ate a particular food, Jane is following a diet plan.

1. The diet is divided into 4 days.
2. The foods are organized according to food family. All members of one family appear on the same day of the diet. A day will be comprised of many food families to cover all the different food groups.

MANAGEMENT

3. The amount of food eaten and the number of times the same food is eaten during the day are not restricted (listen to your own body, it will tell you how much you can handle).
4. Each day includes foods that supply basic nutritional needs.
5. Each day there is a different selection of foods to choose from.

A NOTE ON FOOD FAMILIES:

- An individual will not necessarily be allergic to all members of one family.
- Due to the biological similarities, there is a greater possibility of this occurring, particularly if a different member of the family is eaten every day.

Modifying the Diet:

The diet days as outlined in the pages that follow form a tool to help you control food sensitivity and decrease total body load. They are not carved in stone. Each person will have his or her own list of problem foods. Although they may be written on the choice list, they should still be avoided. By the same token, if a food is listed that you detest, you don't have to eat it. As you work with the diet, you will find ways to make it serviceable for you. Here are some ideas to get you started:

1. Cultural or personal preferences in tastes may be a reason for changing the diet. It is allowed as long as you stay with the concept of biological food families and rotate the families every four days. Setting up the diet, you may move an entire food family to a new day, as long as it becomes a permanent part of that day.
2. You may rearrange the order of the days, however, not sooner than every three months for a child, and at least six months for an adult.

MANAGEMENT

3. Each day represents 24 hours. Instead of beginning your diet day at breakfast, you may start at dinner (allowing you to eat your leftovers for lunch the next day).

4. As you cook, package individual servings in glass jars and freeze for fast meals.

5. Experiment with recipes, play with substitutions.

6. Check your local health food store for acceptable products; there are more and more all the time.

7. Eat organic foods as much as possible.

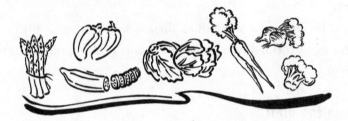

For less sensitive patients, the grass food family is divided into gluten and non-gluten grains eaten on separate days (i.e., day 2 and day 4) to improve food choices.

DAY ONE–FOUR DAY ROTATION DIET

FOOD GROUP	FOOD FAMILY	FOOD FAMILY MEMBERS
FOWL	Pheasant	Chicken and chicken eggs, Cornish hen, pheasant, quail
	Turkey	Turkey
	Duck	Duck and duck eggs, goose and goose eggs
	Emu	Emu
	Ostrich	Ostrich
VEGETABLES	Parsley	Carrot, celeriac (celery root), celery, parsley, parsnip
	Legume	Alfalfa (sprouts), beans (fava, lima, mung & sprouts, navy, white and red kidney beans, black beans, string beans, green and yellow beans), black-eyed pea, green peas, snow peas, chickpea (garbanzo), jicama pea, peanut, soybean, tamarind, tonka bean (courmarin), lentils
	Palm	Palm cabbage
	Yam	Chinese potato (yam)
FRUIT	Laurel	Avocado
	Banana	Banana, plantain
	Palm	Coconut, date
	Pineapple	Pineapple
	Dillenia	Kiwi fruit
	Buckwheat	Rhubarb, sea grape
NUTS/SEEDS	Sapucaya	Brazil nut, paradise nut
	Pedalium	Sesame seeds
GRAIN SUBSTITUTES	Buckwheat	Buckwheat flour, groats
	Legume	Soy, chickpea, lentil flours
STARCHES	Arum	Dasheen arrowroot, taro arrowroot
	Banana	Musa arrowroot
	Legume	Kudzu, carob
	Palm	Sago
OILS	Bird	Bird fat
	Avocado	Avocado
	Legume	Soy, peanut
	Pedalium	Sesame
	Palm	Coconut
FLAVOURINGS	Laurel	Cinnamon, bayleaf, cassia bark, sassafras
	Poppy	Poppyseed
	Pepper	Peppercorns (black and white)
	Borage	Borage, comfrey
	Parsley	Angelica, anise, dill, caraway, celery seed, chervil, coriander, cumin, sweet cicely, fennel, gotu kola, lovage, parsley
	Legume	Fenugreek, licorice, red clover, senna, carob syrup, lecithin, clover honey
	Date	Date sugar
	Buckwheat	Buckwheat honey
OTHER	Buckwheat	Garden sorrel
	Legume	Gum acacia, gum tragacanth, lecithin, soy grits, tofu
	Pedalium	Tahini spread (made from sesame seeds)

MANAGEMENT

DAY TWO–FOUR DAY ROTATION DIET

FOOD GROUP	FOOD FAMILY	FOOD FAMILY MEMBERS
MEAT	Swine	Pork (bacon, ham, lard, pork gelatin, pure pork sausage, scrapple)
	Mollusk	Gastropods (abalone, snail), Cephalopod (squid), Pelecypods (clam, cockle, mussel, oyster, scallop)
	Crustacean	Crab, crayfish, lobster, prawn, shrimp
VEGETABLES	Morning glory	Sweet potato
	Gourd	Chayote, Chinese preserving melon, cucumber, gherkin, pumpkin, squashes (acorn, buttercup, butternut, Boston marrow, crookneck, straight neck, golden nugget, hubbard varieties, spaghetti squash, etc.) zucchini
	Olive	Olives, green and black
	Fungi	Morel, mushroom, puffball, truffle
FRUIT	Cashew	Mango
	Rue (Citrus)	Citron, clementine, grapefruit, kumquat, lemon, lime, mandarin, tangerine, orange, pumello, tangelo, Ugli fruit
	Grape	Grape (brandy, champagne), cream of tartar, raisins, wine, wine vinegar
	Rose berries	Blackberry, boysenberry, dewberry, loganberry, longberry, youngberry, raspberry (black, red, purple), strawberry, wineberry
	Passion Flower	Passion flower fruit (granadilla)
	Gourd	Muskmelons (cantaloupe, casaba, Crenshaw, honeydew, Persian) watermelon
NUTS/SEEDS	Birch	Hazelnut (filbert)
	Cashew	Pistachio, cashew
	Gourd	Pumpkin seeds
GRAINS	Grass*	Corn, millet, rice, teff, sorghum
STARCHES	Grass	Cornstarch
	Morning glory	Sweet potato starch
	Ginger	East Indian arrowroot starch
OILS	Grass	Corn oil
	Olive	Olive oil
	Flax	Flaxseed oil (linseed)
FLAVOURINGS	Citrus	Orange blossom honey
	Ginger	Cardamon, ginger, turmeric
	Grass	Corn syrup, corn sugar,
	Rose Berries	Burnet (herb)
OTHER	Flax	Flaxseed
	Fungi	Baker's yeast, brewer's or nutritional yeast, mold (in certain cheeses)

* gluten-free

DAY THREE–FOUR DAY ROTATION DIET

FOOD GROUP	FOOD FAMILY	FOOD FAMILY MEMBERS
FISH	Herring	Herring, menhaden, sardine, shad
	Salmon	Salmon (all varieties), trout (all freshwater varieties)
	Codfish	Hake, cod, haddock, pollack, whiting
	Roughy	Orange roughy, other types of roughy
	Mackerel	Mackerel, bonito, albacore, tuna
	Flounder	Turbot, halibut, flounder, plaice, sole
	Anchovy	anchovy
VEGETABLES	Mustard	Arugula, broccoli, Brussels sprouts, cabbage, cauliflower, collards, kale, kohlrabi, bok choi, Chinese cabbage, cress (curly, garden, upland, and water) horseradish, mustard greens, mustard seed, radish, rapini, Italian kale, rutabaga, turnip
	Sedge	Water chestnut, groundnut
	Goosefoot	Beet, sugar beet, chard, spinach
	Spurge	Cassava, manioc, mandioca, tapioca
	Brown algae	Kelps(edible seaweed–many species)
	Agave	Agave, aguamiel, yucca
FRUIT	Plum	Apricot, cherry, chokecherry, nectarine, peach, plum
	Blueberry	Blueberry, cranberry, huckleberry
	Mulberry	Mulberry, fig, breadfruit
	Passionflower	Passion fruit
	Soapberry	Litchi
NUTS/SEEDS	Walnut	Black walnut, white walnut (butternut), English walnut, pecan, hickory nut
	Beech	chestnut
GRAIN SUBSTITUTES	Spurge	Cassava (flour)
	Goosefoot	Quinoa (grain and flour)
	Amaranth	Amaranth (seeds and flour)
STARCHES	Spurge	Tapioca starch/flour/pearl
OILS	Mustard	Canola oil (rapeseed)
	Walnut	Walnut oil
	Plum	Almond oil
FLAVOURINGS	Mint	Basil, marjoram, menthol, mint, oregano, peppermint, rosemary, sage, savory, spearmint, thyme
	Myrtle	Allspice, cloves, eucalyptus, feijoa, guava
	Orchid	Vanilla, lychee
	Mustard	Mustard seed
OTHER	Plum	Almond milk and almond butter

MANAGEMENT

DAY FOUR–FOUR DAY ROTATION DIET

FOOD GROUP	FOOD FAMILY	FOOD FAMILY MEMBERS
MEAT	Bovine	Beef, cow's milk, bison (American buffalo), buffalo, ox,
		Goat, goat's milk, sheep, sheep's milk,
		lamb
	Hare	Rabbit
	Deer	Caribou, deer (venison) elk, moose, reindeer
	Opossum	Opossum
	Whale	Whale (all varieties)
	Squirrel	Squirrel
	Bear	Bear
	Horse	Horse
	Pronghorn	Pronghorn
VEGETABLES	Potato	Eggplant, pepino (melon pear), pepper (Anaheim, banana, bell, cherry, chili, jalapeno), tamarillo, tobacco, tomato, tomatillo, white potato
	Lily	Asparagus, aloe, chives, garlic, leek, onion, shallot
	Composite	Dandelion, endive, escarole, Jerusalem artichoke, globe artichoke, lettuce (Boston, iceberg, leaf, Romaine) chicory, radicchio
	Mallow	Okra
FRUIT	Custard apple	Atemoya, custard apple, cherimoya, papaw
	Ebony	Persimmon
	Apple	Apple, loquat, pear, quince
	Papaya	Papaya
	Pomegranate	Pomegranate
	Gooseberry	Gooseberry, true currant
NUTS/SEEDS	Pine	Juniper, pine nuts
	Protea	Macadamia nut
	Composite	Sunflower seeds
GRAINS	Grass*	Barley, kamut, rye, spelt, triticale, oats, Job's tears, wheat
	Composite	Jerusalem Artichoke flour
STARCHES	Potato	Potato starch, potato flour
OILS	Composite	Sunflower oil, safflower oil
	Mallow	Cottonseed oil
	Cattle	Butter
FLAVOURINGS	Composite	Tarragon, burdock, cardoon, chicory, yarrow
	Iris	Saffron
	Lily	Sarsaparilla
	Mallow	Althea root, hibiscus
	Potato	Cayenne pepper, chili, paprika, pimento
	Nutmeg	Nutmeg, mace
OTHER	Apple	Apple cider, apple cider vinegar, rosehip
	Pomegranate	Grenadine
	Composite	Stevia, chamomile, burdock root

* contain gluten

MANAGEMENT

FOR OPTIMUM DIGESTION !!

FOOD COMBINING CHART

- Eat proteins and carbohydrates at separate meals
- Eat only one concentrated protein at each meal
- Treat juices (fruit or vegetable) as whole foods

- Take milk alone or not at all
- Desert desserts
- Cold foods (including liquids) inhibit digestion

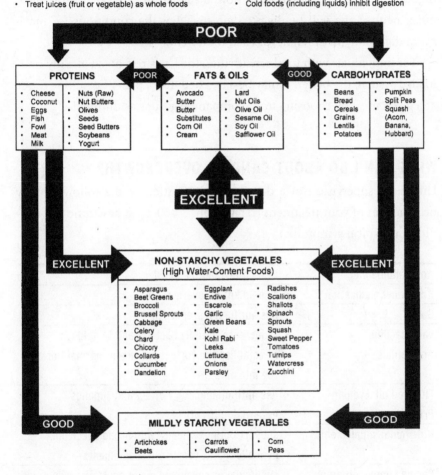

FOOD COMBINING

This method of menu planning involves careful consideration of what food combinations will be digested best by the human system. Within the digestive tract, various digestive juices (enzymes) are excreted to help break down the foods we eat. Different types of food require different enzymes, which in turn function best under enzyme specific conditions. Certain food combinations create conditions that are not compatible, thus reducing the ability to digest the food. For example, protein-rich foods, such as meat, are best digested in an alkaline medium. If both meat and rice are eaten at the same meal, neither one will be digested effectively as the conditions for maximum digestion are different for each food item.

For individuals with food sensitivities, the less stress on an already overloaded system, the better. It may be suggested that a patient combine foods at a given meal by choosing from compatible groups as outlined.

WHAT CAN I DO ABOUT CANDIDA OVERGROWTH?

Under the supervision of a doctor, a combination of the following may become part of your treatment (refer to pp. 69–71 for a description of candida and typical symptoms).

Anti-candida diet	• to stop feeding the yeast
Antifungal medication	• to help kill off overgrowth
Garlic	• has antifungal properties
Lactobacillus Acidophilus	• to increase friendly bacteria and to help re-establish the correct balance or normal flora in the intestine
Flaxseed oil, Evening Primrose oil	• has anti-inflammatory effect and supplies essential nutrients
Nutritional supplements	• support optimum health with broad spectrum, hypoallergenic, yeast-free supplements
Candida immunotherapy	• sublingual or subcutaneous to neutralize symptoms from Candida
Reduction of total body load	• avoid or control other sensitivities (e.g., allergenic foods), decrease stress level, exercise

MANAGEMENT

Beat the Yeast

For individuals with mold sensitivities and yeast problems, controlling the intake of certain foods is essential for improvement. There are many versions of the yeast free diet, some more restrictive than others. The following is a general summary of foods to be avoided. Please remember that no two individuals are alike, and your own sensitivities must be kept in mind when applying this information to your rotation diet.

Avoid:

| Sweeteners | Yeasts | Fermented Products | Vinegar | Pickled & Smoked Foods | Moldy Foods |

Avoiding sweeteners

- avoid refined sugars (date, cane, beet, corn and fruit)
- you may tolerate in moderation fresh fruit, honey (maximum of one teaspoon per day)

Avoiding yeast

- avoid commercial baker's yeast
- avoid brewer's yeast
- avoid nutritional supplements containing yeast
- you may tolerate breads baked with sourdough as leavener; sourdough is wild yeast and a bacterial culture.

Avoiding fermented products

- avoid ciders, soy sauce, alcohol, root beer, miso

MANAGEMENT

Avoiding vinegar

- avoid salad dressings, mayonnaise, mustard, ketchup, sauces

Avoiding pickled and smoked foods

- avoid relish, pickles and pickled vegetables, smoked fish and meat

Avoiding moldy foods

- avoid mushrooms, leftovers, aged cheeses
- avoid fruits that are prone to mold, e.g., cantaloupes and grapes
- avoid dried fruits unless they are mold-free

Food for thought

- Fruit juices ferment easily. Use freshly made vegetable and fruit juice and consume quickly.
- Clean your vegetables well before storing them. Store in the fridge but not too long. Better to buy smaller quantities, more often.
- Buy nuts raw and roast at home. 350-degree oven for 10-20 minutes.
- Cook all root vegetables after peeling and washing.
- Watch out for mold growth when purchasing foods.
- Antibiotics, steroids, both oral and topical, chemotherapy, radiation, immunosuppressive medications such as methotrexate and azothioprine, and starvation, all contribute to the development of yeast.

NUTRITIONAL SUPPLEMENTS

Vitamins, Minerals, Amino Acids

How often we hear: "If you eat a balanced diet you do not need to take supplements." Some individuals and most doctors do not "believe in" supplements. However, this approach to health is not about religion. Supplementation is based on science.

MANAGEMENT

RDAs or Recommended Daily Allowances (in Canada called Recommended Nutrient Intakes or RNIs) were established by the Food and Nutrition Board of the National Academy of Sciences/National Research Council in the US and are based on requirements for nutrients needed to metabolize foods equivalent to 2000 calories for women and 3000 calories for men.

Diets based on RDAs do not consider:

I Individual lifestyle:

- The busy worker or executive has no time to calculate intake of protein, carbohydrates and fats.
- The overworked teacher doesn't know how much complex carbohydrate to take.
- Carefree teenagers or tired seniors do not know how much protein is in cheese.

II Poor availability of all nutrients from our diets due to:

- Food preferences: overeating some products, ignoring others
- Habits – level of appetite, dieting, fast foods, packaged foods
- Food availability: lower income = less availability
- Loss of nutrients through:

Storage: – Fruits and vegetables are picked, stored, shipped and stored again

– $2/3$ of vitamin C lost from apples in 2 months

– vegetables lose all their vitamin C within a few days

– oranges lose 30% of vitamin C when squeezed

– No vitamin C in commercial juices unless added back in

Processing: heat, light water, chemicals (e.g., "enriched" white bread, is refined "dead food" to which a few token supplements have been added back)

Blanching: of vegetables before freezing: 60% loss of vitamin C, 30% loss of B_1, 40% loss of B_2

Sterilization: Irradiation causes a 69% loss of vitamins

Cooking: 50% loss of vitamins

Milling of grains: 40% loss of vitamin C, 65-80% loss of all B vitamins, 59% loss of magnesium, 72% loss of zinc

Intensive industrial farming: Pesticides, fertilizers, lack of crop rotation, acid rain, all lead to degradation of soil and a lower content of minerals. Loss of zinc, selenium, magnesium, calcium automatically increases the content of heavy metals in the soil.

Fertilization: speeds growth and decreases relative content of nutrients.

III Biochemical individuality (one size will not fit all)

- We are all unique and require different amounts of nutrients
- Documented inborn errors of metabolism can increase requirements for specific nutrients by 10-100 times
- Pollution of water, air and food requires more nutrients (antioxidants) to metabolize the pollutants
- Psychological stress of daily living calls for more nutrients
- Diseases interfering with digestion, absorption, assimilation and repair: Celiac, Crohn's, ulcerative colitis, lactose intolerance, bacterial, viral, parasitic infections, trauma, burns, surgery, all require more nutrients
- Drugs: antibiotics, diuretics, contraceptive pills, antidepressants, steroids, alcohol, all decrease nutrients
- Aging: organs function less efficiently and cause decreased digestion and absorption.

Optimum health

Vitamins and minerals are used in every metabolic step and process in our bodies. Overt disease from a lack of specific nutrients, e.g., scurvy (C), rickets

(D), anemia (B$_{12}$), beri-beri (B$_1$), indicates its end-stage. Before this stage occurs, there has been a steady reduction in the body's store of nutrients. This leads to a depletion of enzymes, which depend on vitamins and minerals and finally, cells cannot perform their function. This intermediate stage is called **subclinical nutrient deficiency,** which is chronic and predisposes the individual to:

- reduced overall health and quality of life
- decreased ability to cope with life stresses
- premature aging
- weakening of the immune, neurological and endocrine systems
- triggering development of genetically inherited illnesses such as diabetes, cancer, cardiac diseases, allergies

RDAs are the nutritional equivalent of the minimum wage. Diets based on them will keep us alive, but not functioning at an optimum level of health and quality of life. It would be better to change RDAs to ODAs, or Optimal Daily Allowances.

For these reasons, while it is always best to obtain and assimilate all needed vitamins, minerals and enzymes from fresh, living, organic food, the fact is that most of us do not. Therefore, supplementation is recommended.

Doses depend on the condition and needs of the individual. It is usually best to take supplements with food (particularly B vitamins, which may cause nausea if taken alone), in divided doses throughout the day. Natural source is preferable to synthetic. Gel capsules are better than tablets. Some individuals cannot tolerate some vitamins. Excipients may be the problem in these cases. Look for hypoallergenic brands (free of yeast, wheat, corn, sugar, milk, soy). B vitamins in gelatin capsule form might be better tolerated. Experiment until you find the right one for you. A doctor or holistic practitioner using an electrodermal instrument can help you find a well-tolerated supplement.

AMINO ACIDS

Amino acids are:

- building blocks of peptides (hormones such as human growth hormone [HGH], insulin, thymus hormone, etc.) and proteins (enzymes, all organs)
- precursors for many neurotransmitters (tryptophan → serotonin, phenylalanine → norepinephrine, tyrosine → dopamine, etc.)

In combination with vitamins and minerals, they are used to successfully manage and help many chronic and degenerative diseses. They may be used orally or intravenously to restore health. If used, most need a high dose of at least 2-3 + gms per day ("L-" forms must be used). Some stimulate secretion of the individual's own growth hormone, which in turn increases metabolism in the entire body.

Any use requires ruling out, and treatment of, any underlying infections (stealth infections, see page 292) as well as assessment of prolactin, which is the marker for a pituitary tumour (one in four, more female than male persons, may have this tumour), which would be a contraindication for use of amino acids stimulating the growth hormone.

Keeping in mind that appropriate vitamins and minerals should be added in combination, following are some examples of the clinical use of amino acids:

Central Nervous System:

- **Anxiety:** Glutamine; Glutamic Acid; Glycine; Taurine; GABA
  Exercise → ↑ GABA, ↑ dopamine, ↑ endorphins
- **Depression:** Phenylalanine; Tyrosine; Tryptophan; Leucine; Treonine
- **Epilepsy:** Taurine; Glutamine; Arginine; Aspartic Acid; GABA
- **Memory:** Phosphatidylcholine PC; Phosphatidylserine PS
- **Multiple Sclerosis (MS):** Serine; Treonine; Tryptophan; Choline
- **Parkinson's:** Phenylalanine; Tyrosine; Taurine; Glutathione

Gastrointestinal System
- **Ammonia Removal:** Glutamic Acid; Lysine; Aspartic Acid; Asparagine; Ornitine
- **Cravings/Addictions:** Glutamine; Glycine; Serine; Alanine; Salsolinol; Chromium
- **Dysbiosis:** Glutamine; Glycine; Taurine; Treonine
- **Gallstones/Sludge:** Taurine

Other
- **Detoxification for Chemicals, Heavy Metals, Radiation:** Methionine (precursor to Cystein and Cystine); Taurine; Glutathione
- **Chronic Fatigue:** Arginine; Leucine; Isoleucine; Alanine; Glycine; Glutamine; Tryptophan
- **Immune Stimulation:** Arginine; Asparagine; Aspartic Acid; Serine; Treonine; Taurine
- **Arthritis:** Proline; Treonine; Methionine
- **Congestive Heart/Arrythmias:** Taurine; Proline
- **Hair, Nails, Skin:** Lysine; Methionine; Taurine
- **Viruses:** Lysine; Glycine

MANAGEMENT

MANAGEMENT

MINERAL	DEFICIENCY MARKER	FOOD SOURCE	ASSIMILATION AIDS	ASSIMILATION BARRIERS	RDA*	ODA**
Calcium Ca *Macro element*	Muscle cramps & tremors, joint pain, arthritis, rickets, osteoporosis, osteomalacia, tooth decay, insomnia, nervousness	Milk products, sesame seeds, almonds, sardines, salmon	Vitamins A, C, D, Boron, Magnesium. Best in calcium magnesium ratio of 2:1	Refined sugar & flour, additives, toxic metals, processed foods, coffee, tea, alcohol, carbonated drinks. Aluminum, lead	1200 mg	1500 mg
Magnesium Mg *Macro element*	Muscle cramps, tremors, weakness, insomnia, anxiety, depression, high blood pressure, arrhythmias, PMS, convulsions, hyperactivity, constipation	Wheat germ, brewer's yeast, nuts, almonds, cashews, brazil nuts, dairy foods, meat, fish, cocoa	Vitamins B6, C, D, Zinc, Calcium, Phosphorus	Excess milk products, fats, oxalates (spinach & rhubarb), alcohol, diuretics	280-350 mg	500-700 mg
Phosphorus P *Macro element*	Appetite loss, fatigue, weak bones, teeth, joint problems	Available in most foods, meat, dairy. Sodas can be very high and lead to health problem.	Calcium	Antacids Aluminum	800 mg	800 mg

Element	Deficiency symptoms	Food sources	Synergists	Depleters		
Potassium K *Macro element*	Arrhythmias, ↑ blood pressure, nervous disorders, muscle weakness, constipation, nausea, cellulite	Molasses, dates, parsley, banana, cauliflower, pumpkin, dairy, meat, poultry, fish	Magnesium, sodium, B6	Diuretics, laxatives, corticosteroids, salt in excess, alcohol, smoking, tea, coffee	None noted	100-300 mg
Sodium Na *Macro element*	Nausea, dizziness, weakness, low blood pressure, mental apathy, muscle cramps	Salt, olives, celery, cabbage, seafood	Vitamin D, Potassium	Diuretics	None noted	2400 mg
Iron Fe *Macro element*	Anemia, fatigue, brittle nails, breathing difficulties	Molasses, eggs, fish, organ meats, pumpkin seeds, dark green vegetables	Vitamin C, B1, folic acid	Oxalates (spinach, rhubarb), tannic acid (tea)	10-15 mg	15-30 mg
Zinc Zn *Macro element*	↓ smell & taste, delayed maturity, slow wound healing, slow growth, prostate enlargement, ↓ immunity	Oysters, fish, seafood, whole grains, poultry, mushrooms, legumes	Good stomach acid, Vitamin B6, calcium, magnesium	Phytates (e.g., wheat), oxalates, excess copper, diuretics. Lead, aluminum, cadmium, mercury.	18-12 mg	20-50 mg

MANAGEMENT

MANAGEMENT

MINERAL	DEFICIENCY MARKER	FOOD SOURCE	ASSIMILATION AIDS	ASSIMILATION BARRIERS	RDA*	ODA**
Boron B *Trace element*	Osteoporosis	Most fruits and vegetables	Balanced vitamin & mineral intake	Unknown	None noted	3-6 mg
Chromium Cr *Trace element*	Glucose metabolism disorders, cravings, cold sweats, dizziness, drowsiness, irritability, thirst, cold hands	Brewer's yeast, whole grains, herbs and spices	Vitamin B3, amino acids (glycine, glutamine, cystine)	Refined sugars and flour	10-25 mcg	200-600 mcg
Cobalt Co *Trace element*	Pernicious anemia, central & peripheral neurological disturbances	Green leafy vegetables, organ meats, brewer's yeast	Vitamin B12, folic acid	Unknown	None noted	8 mcg
Copper Cu *Trace element*	Loss of lung elasticity (emphysema), collagen disorders, anemia	Legumes, nuts, seeds, organ meats, whole grains, mushrooms, cocoa, copper pans and pipes	Cobalt, iron, zinc	Excess zinc, mercury, cadmium.	1 mg	2 mg

	Deficiency symptoms	Food sources		Causes / antagonists		
Iodine I *Trace element*	Thyroid disorders, cystic breast disease	Sea food, saltwater fish, kelp, iodized salt	None	Too many cruciferous vegetables (e.g., cabbage, broccoli, cauliflower)	150 mcg	Up to 300 mcg
Manganese Mn *Trace element*	Ataxia (muscle coordination failure), ↓ hearing, ear buzzing, ringing, growing pains	Whole grains, eggs, organ meats, green leafy vegetables, legumes	None	Refined foods, alcohol, tea, coffee, antibiotics	None noted	5-10 mg
Selenium Se *Trace element*	Increased rates of cancer and heart disease. Premature aging, hair loss	Organ meats, seafood, plants (depending on soil selenium content)	Vitamins A, C, E	Refined foods, modern farming techniques. cadmium, mercury.	55-70 mcg	50-400 mcg

MANAGEMENT

VITAMIN	DEFICIENCY MARKER	FOOD SOURCE	ASSIMILATION AIDS	ASSIMILATION BARRIERS	RDA*	ODA**
Vitamin A Retinol & betacarotene *Fat soluble*	Mouth ulcers, acne, ↓ night vision, macular degeneration, ↑ infections, dandruff, dry skin, thrush, cystitis, insomnia	Green & yellow fruits & vegetables, eggs, milk products, liver, fish oil	Zinc, Vit C & E, C, multivitamin. Taken with food	Heat, light, alcohol, coffee, smoking, antibiotics, laxatives	4000-5000 IU	10,000-75,000 IU
B1 Thiamine *Water soluble*	Nervous system disease, ↓ memory, concentration, muscle, eye pain, digestive disturbances, appetite loss, fatigue	Brewer's yeast, molasses, unrefined grains, brown rice, nuts, fish, meat, poultry, beans	Other B vitamins, magnesium, manganese. Taken with food	Antibiotics, alcohol, tea, coffee, stress, birth control pills	1.2-1.4 mg	25-300 mg
B2 Riboflavin *Water soluble*	Burning, gritty eyes, cataracts, light sensitivity, cracks & sores in mouth corners, split nails, dull, oily hair, eczema	Brewer's yeast, molasses, nuts, whole grains, egg yolk, green leafy vegetables, fish, poultry, meat, nuts, beans	Other B vitamins, selenium. Taken with food	Alcohol, birth control pills, tea, coffee, antibiotics	1.2-1.4 mg	25-300 mg

	Deficiency symptoms	Food sources	Synergists	Depleted by	RDA	Dosage
B3 Niacin *Water soluble*	Fatigue, headaches, insomnia, anxiety, depression, poor memory, bleeding gums, acne, pellagra (3 Ds: dermatitis, dementia, diarrhea)	Brewer's yeast, seafood, fish, milk products, poultry, peanuts, whole grains, sesame seeds, mushrooms	Other B vitamins, chromium. Taken with food	Anitibiotics, tea, coffee, oral contraceptives, alcohol	1.2-1.4 mg	25-300 mg
B5 Pantothenic Acid *Water soluble*	Adrenal insufficiency, fatigue, muscle tremors, cramps, burning feet, tender heels, apathy, ↓ endurance, nausea	Brewer's yeast, legumes, organ meats, whole grains, eggs, green vegetables, salmon, mushrooms	Other B vitamins, Vitamin C, biotin, folic acid. Taken with food	Stress, alcohol, tea, coffee	None noted	25-300 mg
B6 Pyridoxine *Water soluble*	Water retention, tingling hands, joint problems, muscle tremors, cramps, acne, anemia, depression, irritability	Brewer's yeast, molasses, bananas, green vegetables, beans, eggs, meats, whole grains	Other B vitamins, zinc, magnesium, potassium. Taken with food	Alcohol, smoking, oral contraceptives, antidepressants, food processing, cooking	1.2-1.4 mg	25-300 mg
B12 Cyanocobalamin *Water soluble*	Anxiety, depression, fatigue, poor hair condition, dermatitis, anemia	Brewer's yeast, organ meats, sardines, fish, milk products	Folic acid, other B vitamins. Taken with food	Alcohol, smoking, low stomach acid, anticoagulants, food processing, cooking	2 mcg	25-300 mcg

MANAGEMENT

MANAGEMENT

VITAMIN	DEFICIENCY MARKER	FOOD SOURCE	ASSIMILATION AIDS	ASSIMILATION BARRIERS	RDA*	ODA**
Biotin *Water soluble*	Dry skin, baldness, premature graying, fatigue, muscle pain, insomnia	Eggs, almonds, lettuce, poultry, yeast, soybeans, whole grains	B vitamins, magnesium, manganese. Taken with food	Fried foods, antibiotics, sulpha drugs, saccharin	None noted	25-300 mcg
Folic acid *Water soluble*	Anemia, premature graying, anxiety, poor memory, fatigue, depression, growth problems, fetal neural tube defects, cervical dysplasia	Green leafy vegetables, milk products, organ meats, lentils, sesame seeds, wheat germ, peanuts	B vitamins especially B12. Taken with food	Food processing, cooking, oral contraceptives, alcohol, smoking	150-200 mcg	400-1200 mcg
Vitamin C Ascorbic Acid *Water soluble*	Frequent colds & infections, ↓ immunity, ↑ cholesterol & blood pressure, bleeding gums & nose, bruising, fatigue, anemia, slow wound healing, collagen tissue disorders, ↓ adrenal function	Berries, black currants, citrus, sauerkraut, tropical fruits, peppers, broccoli	Bioflavinoids, all B vitamins (to produce energy), Vitamin E (as antioxidant)	Smoking, oral contraceptives, alcohol, pollution, stress, antidepressants	60 mg	500-5000 mg and higher if under stress

	Deficiency symptoms	Sources	Depleted by	Works with	RDA*	ODA**
Vitamin D Calciferol *Fat soluble*	Rickets, softening bones & teeth, osteoporosis, muscle spasms, insomnia, hair loss, depression, ↓ immunity	Fish oils, herring, mackerel, eggs, fortified dairy products	Lack of sunlight	Exposure to sunlight, calcium, vitamins A, C	400 IU	400–1000 IU up to 2000 IU in winter
Vitamin E Tocopherols *Fat soluble*	Cardiovascular disorders, infertility, ↓ sex drive, PMS, dry skin, gastrointestinal problems, muscular wasting	Cold-pressed vegetable oils, whole grains, green vegetables, nuts, legumes, sunflower & sesame seeds, wheat germ	High cooking temperature, oral contraceptives, air pollution	Vitamin C, selenium, zinc, copper, phosphorous	8–10 IU	200–800 IU
Vitamin K Phytomenadione *Fat soluble*	Blood clotting problems, osteoporosis	Green leafy vegetables, organ meats, cauliflower, brussels sprouts, legumes	Antibiotics	Healthy intestinal bacteria, breastfeeding for babies	65–80 mcg	Not determined

* RDA-Recommended Daily Allowance (as set by US Food & Nutrition Boards) : these are minimum requirements

** ODA-Optimal Daily Allowance : for optimal health

Both RDA and ODA are age, gender and physiological state (e.g., pregnancy) dependent

Physicians practicing Orthomolecular medicine may prescribe higher doses for therapeutic reasons

MANAGEMENT

INTRAVENOUS USE OF NUTRIENTS

There are well-developed protocols and specific indications for use of intravenous therapies. They include:

- Acute viral infections, when use of antibiotics has no significant value
- Acute or chronic debilitating fatigue
- Bacterial infections, for the purpose of protecting cells from toxicity due to concurrent antibiotic use
- Major surgery, both before and after to improve wound healing
- Chemotherapy, before and after to protect cells from cytotoxic injury
- Chemical toxicity (Multiple Chemical Sensitivity) to overcome enzymatic blockage which prevents nutrients from entering metabolic pathways
- Heavy metal toxicity
- Malabsorption related to food, mold allergies, candida overgrowth, parasitic infestations, various inflammatory bowel diseases such as ulcerative colitis, etc.
- Intravenous use can be important in the very ill patient, where nutrients need to be directed immediately to the organ in need
- Some patients can only tolerate one or two vitamins at first, but can develop tolerance as treatment progresses
- Preservative-free vitamins and mineral solutions are recommended
- Often required on a basis of once or twice per week for 5 to 10 weeks and then only when required

CHELATION THERAPY

Chelation therapy with EDTA, DMPS and DMSA is indicated for heavy metal toxicity. Chelation therapy with EDTA is indicated for atherosclerotic cardiovascular disease in order to reverse atherosclerotic coronary and peripheral lesions. This requires specific protocols in consideration of individual weight, height and medical condition. Physicians who are members of the American College for Advancement in Medicine (ACAM) have training and experience in using these protocols. You can get more information in books written on the subject, such as *Bypassing Bypass Surgery: The New Technique of Chelation Therapy*, by Elmer Cranton, M.D.; Hampton Roads Publishing Company, 1992. Conditions which can be helped significantly by chelation therapy include:

- Advanced atherosclerosis of cerebral vascular insufficiency (confused, tired, poor memory, fainting, dizziness, etc.)
- Coronary artery diseases: angina, post heart attacks, post bypass surgery and angioplasty (conditions which can often be prevented by early institution of EDTA chelation therapy)

MANAGEMENT

- Peripheral artery disease: pain in upper or lower extremities due to arterial insufficiency, stroke
- Hypertension, high cholesterol, diabetes
- Alzheimer's disease, scleroderma
- Healthy individuals—to prevent the onset of age-associated vascular disease before symptoms occur

(See Appendix)

Special Interest

ATTENTION DEFICIT HYPERACTIVE DISORDER (ADHD)

Attention Deficit Hyperactive Disorder (ADHD) is a condition that causes many problems throughout life and is not restricted to children. It is a growing problem for which allopathic medicine has neither a recognizable cause nor an effective treatment. It is not only a problem for the individual diagnosed with ADHD, but also causes anguish and worry for family members, and difficulty for educators. Many books are available on this topic, but one of the best continues to be *Is This Your Child's World?*, by Dr. Doris Rapp, Bantam Books 1996. Dr. Rapp is a traditional pediatric allergist, who has used the principles of Environmental Medicine for over thirty years. She combines the knowledge of the two disciplines and presents a comprehensive and useful guide for parents and educators, as well as successful treatment options for many ADD children.

The last twenty years have not improved the recognition or the management of ADHD. The approved treatment for ADHD is still very much drug-oriented. What has changed are the names used for labeling this disorder. In the last twenty years, such terms as hyperactivity, hyperkineses, minimal brain dysfunction and attention span deficiency syndrome have been applied. Today it is referred to as Attention Deficit Hyperactive Disorder and in some more severe cases, the term Pervasive Developmental Disorder (PDD) is used.

Over this time span, there has emerged a great pressure by physicians, daycare providers, and educators to place these children on an activity-modifying class II narcotic with the trade name of Ritalin. In some cases, parents are threatened and even forced to comply with the recommendation to place their children on Ritalin, or they are left with the option of seeking alternate school accommodation. Approximately eight million children in the US take Ritalin.

Exact statistics on the number of children with ADHD are not available due to confusion with other related disorders. For example, 66% of ADHD-diagnosed children have hidden unrecognized food allergies that are responsible for many symptoms common to both disorders. Other children's behaviour may be affected dramatically when exposed to dust, molds and chemicals. In a survey taken by the American Academy of Pediatrics, 71% of teachers stated that they see more and more health problems, and up to 20% of US children have chronic health conditions (American Academy of Pediatrics, School Health Policy and Practice, 1993).

It is estimated that at least 10% of school children suffer from ADHD, therefore, in a normal class size of thirty children, three will present with ADHD. The ratio of boys to girls is four to one. It is interesting to note that a majority of children with ADHD have signs and symptoms related to environmental illness as described on pp. 38–39 in the earlier chapters of this guide.

Typical Characteristics of ADHD
- Short attention span
- Easily distracted
- Overactive and disoriented
- Disturbing other children
- Not able to sit still

- Impulsive, sometimes violent
- Dull appearance or day dreamer
- Emotional problems, easily crying, depressed
- Discipline problems
- Poor coordination
- Perceptual problems

Resultant Problems

- Listening
- Thinking
- Talking, reading or spelling
- Writing
- Arithmetic

} depending on which difficulty or combination of difficulties will contribute to the level of **learning disability**

Parents and educators should know that the **signs and symptoms of children with ADHD change** as they progress in age:

Prenatal

With many children, their mothers could feel excessive movements in utero—hiccups, painful kicking or worrisome quiet. These symptoms would be noticed a few minutes after ingestion of an allergic food to which the fetus had become sensitized in utero. Often the culprit is milk consumed excessively by the mother, since women are encouraged to "drink milk," especially when pregnant.

Infancy

At this stage, the baby may cry and scream excessively, have colic, which leads to frequent formula changes, and have difficulty sleeping (difficulty falling asleep and waking up frequently). They may present with eczema, constant nasal stuffiness and/or a runny nose. They may suffer from chronic ear infections. There is a lot of drooling and excessive perspiration, and as they get a bit older, they rock and bang their head against the crib.

SPECIAL INTEREST

Toddler

In the toddler stage, ADHD children are not able to cuddle. They constantly wiggle, exhibit excessive temper tantrums, may bite self or others, and often take their clothes off. Some sleep a lot (child narcolepsy), have one cold after another, repeated ear infections leading to chronic use of antibiotics, and complain of leg pain, which is described in pediatric literature as "growing pains." (In my experience and opinion, no healthy child should experience leg pain. A simple elimination of allergic food, and particularly food dyes, often cures these children of leg pain completely.)

Preschool

The preschool child's symptoms change to chronic runny noses and stuffiness, and ultimately the "salute crease" or "allergic wipe" (constantly rubbing the nose upward, which leaves the nose with a permanent crease). Breathing problems, such as bronchitis and/or the beginnings of asthma, start. Other gastrointestinal symptoms begin: diarrhea, constipation, excessive gas, abdominal pain, bad breath, and rushing to the bathroom. Excessive tiredness or hyperactivity is observed and learning problems begin. It is often a teacher who observes this first and informs the parents about the problem.

Adolescence

As time passes and the physiology changes in adolescence, these children show a different picture. Chronic tiredness sets in, muscle pain, headaches could be troublesome; emotional instability, irritability, forgetfulness, and inability to think clearly could be another set of symptoms. At this age, some eat excessively and become obese, while others develop anorexia. They feel inadequate, tired, and often turn to drugs or alcohol. Depression and suicidal tendency is common. What is interesting is that often their previous eczema or asthma may disappear due to the surge of steroid hormones as a result of their sexual development. This is misleading to parents, as poorly informed doctors tell parents that the children have outgrown their previous problems. This "outgrowing phenomenon" misconception is falsely comforting to parents. This theory was discussed on p. 38 under the title Changing Faces of Sensitivity.

Cause of ADHD

The causes of ADHD are not clear, and sometimes controversial. A well-accepted hypothesis is low oxygen or hypoxia of the brain as a result of difficulties in labour, such as breech delivery, cord wrapped around the infants neck, compression of the umbilical cord in the birth canal, or prolapse of the umbilical cord. Stress and lack of oxygen produce infants with abnormalities in their appearance, respiration and heart rate at birth. Their APGAR score in the first and even second minute after delivery is low (a perfect APGAR score is 10 in the first minute).

Other possible causes of ADHD are viral or bacterial meningitis in early childhood, intoxication in utero with lead, mercury or other heavy metals, anemias of different origin, and undetected hypothyroidism (low function of the thyroid) and lack of early treatment. Any form of physical, mental or sexual abuse can also affect a child's learning and behaviour.

One disturbing hypothesis based on numerous animal studies (but limited human studies) is the theory that persistent chemicals are able to inhibit the action of thyroid hormones that are crucial for developing brain intelligence. The chemicals referred to in this theory are the hormone-disrupting chlorinated pesticides and plastics, particularly PCBs. Considering the continuous and widespread use of these chemicals globally, this problem could have catastrophic consequences on the development of our children and the ability of future generations to conduct intelligent life and activity on this earth.

In my own environmental practice, I see an alarming number of children with ADHD. Most parents come armed with pages of documentation regarding their child's condition, and they are not satisfied with their child's progress on the traditional treatment. After appropriate testing, we find that a large majority of these children are affected by other environmental and dietary factors. Food allergy and sensitivity, chemical toxicity

SPECIAL INTEREST

and chemical sensitivity, and mold, dust, dust mite and other inhalant allergies will be evident. Some of the ADHD children have vitamin, mineral and essential fatty acid deficiencies when they first come to see me. Early recognition and treatment of these allergies and deficiencies could bring relief to thousands of children with ADHD, allowing them to discontinue Ritalin or use a very minimal dose.

There are many environmental offenders at home and in schools that can be changed to help improve ADHD. Once parents are made aware of some environmental controls at home that can improve their child's behaviour (e.g., removing scented products, using air cleaners, dust mite covers for mattresses, etc., as previously directed in the Management section, they are generally put into place. Dealing with schools and school boards is not always that simple.

Sick building syndrome problems related to schools have a profound effect on the health and learning of our children. A report by the Occupational Safety and Health Administration showed that over 50% (15 out of 29 state universities) had air quality problems, of which 73% qualified as sick building syndrome. Airborne chemicals were contributing to the trouble of the buildings in 63% in the same study (American Academy of Pediatrics School Health: Policy and Practice 1993).

The school environment and how it can impact the health of an environmentally sensitive child has been discussed in the Management section on page 202. The same recommendations could be applied to significantly improve the health and behaviour of ADHD children.

Nutrition plays an important role in treating children with ADHD. Keeping them off their allergenic foods helps considerably, but keeping them away from "junk food" is just as important. This is not an easy task, considering the persuasive television advertising and the number of fast food outlets cropping up. "Junk food" contains many chemicals that have detrimental effects on the brains of these children.

Lack of physical exercise, lack of art and music programs because of funding cuts, as well as excessive time spent in front of television and computer screens watching or playing questionable violent shows or games, all contribute to learning disabilities and behaviour problems at home, school or in society at large.

What can be done?

- A thorough environmental history should be taken. Looking for a cause will help to individualize the treatment. The mother's history, including time of pregnancy, occupation during pregnancy, geographical location and activities during pregnancy, are all important. Basic laboratory tests to rule out simple causes such as like anemia or hypothyroidism should be performed. Psychological testing is very important, as well as hearing and visual assessments. Further specialized tests for detection of heavy metals, and tests to detect vitamin, mineral and essential fatty acid deficiencies should be performed. Food, chemical and inhalant allergies and/or sensitivities should be determined by either sublingual, intradermal or electrodermal testing (or ELISA tests on blood) as described earlier in this guide.

- Once allergies are determined, environmental controls should be implemented at home and in the school. This may require education on the part of the parents and the educators and superintendents of the school (refer to section on Indoor Air Pollution, and the School Environment).

- Change of diet with elimination of all allergic foods, and especially "junk food," and introduction of the four-day rotation diet is necessary for at least three months (see Four-Day Rotation Diet, p. 222).

- Nutritional supplementation of vitamins and minerals, especially B vitamins and zinc, together with essential fatty acids, is a must in all cases of ADHD. Some herbal preparations such as ADFX, containing an extract of Ginko Biloba and American Ginseng, may have some value in treating ADHD also. Addition of Phosphatidylcholine and Phosphatidylserine, along with Ginko Biloba, may be very important to increase the activity of the parasympathetic system and increase CNS circulation.

SPECIAL INTEREST

- Food, chemical and inhalant sensitivities should be treated in addition to environmental controls with desensitization in the form of sublingual neutralizing drops or Enzyme Potentiated Desensitization (EPD).
- Children with ADHD may benefit from special education classes where the ratio of teacher to student is much smaller. Four or six children to one teacher is ideal.
- An ADHD child will improve and benefit faster if all members of the family adhere to the environmental controls and the four-day rotation diet.

In the majority of cases, this approach gives excellent results, and the need for Ritalin is diminished. Children concentrate better, their activity level settles down, they improve healthwise, and they regain their much-needed self-esteem. Some children may still require Ritalin, but the above-mentioned recommendations allow the effective dose of Ritalin to be greatly reduced.

Since we know that ADHD can be influenced in the womb, prevention can begin before conception and during pregnancy. All women of child-bearing age should avoid working in contaminated places where chemicals, plastics, and toxins are present. They should stop smoking and drinking alcohol and coffee long before conception. Perhaps special education regarding the importance of a nutritious diet, avoidance of persistent chemicals in the environment and the workplace, and maintaining overall good health should be implemented during high school years, and stressed to both young men and women.

During pregnancy, women (especially if they are aware of allergies in their family) should stay on a four-day rotation diet, and optimally eat organic foods. This is advisable for both the time of pregnancy and breastfeeding, which is recommended to continue to at least one year of age. Introduction of foods is covered in the section on Infants on page 265.

SPECIAL INTEREST

AUTISM

Autism, also called Pervasive Developmental Disorder (PDD) or Autistic Spectrum Disorder, is a rapidly increasing disorder in North America, Europe and Asia, a fact noticed in the early 80s. Today, in the US, one in every 160 school-aged children suffers from it. It is more prevalent in boys (one in eighty in the US has autism nationwide and one in fifty in England). In spite of the common belief that autism is a psychological/psychiatric disorder, recent data indicate that it is more a biological problem.

For many years, there was little research into autism or help for autistic children and their families. In 1995, Dr. Bernard Rimland (the father of an autistic son) and his Autism Research Institute, established in 1967, began to convene regular conferences for interested physicians and scientists, as well as parents under the name DAN! (Defeat Autism Now!) with the purpose of sharing research, information, ideas and working toward the goal of finding effective treatments.

Over the years, the DAN! Protocol has been developed, which guides physicians and parents to clinical assessment options leading to appropriate treatment. This protocol is of interest, particularly to parents and physicians who do not consider psychotropic drugs as the best or only choice of treatment. Briefly:

Detailed history with a view to possible causative factors, including:
- Intoxication with toxic chemicals, heavy metals
- Vaccination problems
- Birth injury
- Signs and symptoms of allergies/sensitivities
- History of infections
- Specific organ disorders such as dysbiosis.

Testing includes:
- Iron level (to rule out anemia)
- Ammonia level (> 70% autistic children have elevated levels from dysbiosis due to overgrowth of fungus, bacteria or parasites)
- Oxidative stress
- Antioxidant, amino acids, essential oil levels
- Organic acids
- Age-dependent 24-hour urinalysis for mercury and other heavy metals
- Allergy/sensitivity screening

Depending on results of tests, treatments may include:
- Casein-free and gluten-free diet
- Allergy desensitization
- Nutritional therapy
- Detoxification through supplements
- Chelation for heavy metals
- Sauna
- Metabolic correction
- Secretin injections every 6 weeks
- Behavioural modification

Many parents with autistic children have already discovered that removing milk products (casein/caseomorphin) and gluten products (gliadomorphin) from the child's diet brings the most effective improvement in behaviour and general health. Most parents already involve the child in behaviour modification or Applied Behaviour Analysis (ABA).

Allergies and sensitivities can best be managed with Enzyme Potentiated Desensitization (EPD), which offers the broadest desensitization umbrella for food, inhalants, molds, bacteria, etc. EPD and concomitant therapy allows for appropriate nutrition with minerals, vitamins, magnesium, zinc, and also systematically treats dysbiosis. A prolonged anti-candida treatment, if necessary, can be given between EPD shots. If underlying problems are of an immune or autoimmune nature, use of immune modulators such as colostrum or thymus extract may be indicated. Any dental mercury amalgams should be replaced.

All supplements should be hypoallergenic and screened for tolerance by electrodermal method (the easiest under the circumstances). Mercury-free products only, i.e., no fish or fish oils.

Autism is a multi-disciplinary problem involving toxicology, epidemiology, neurology, immunology, genetics, gastroenterology, etc. There is no one answer for any autistic child. Parent and doctor work together to determine contributing factors and try various researched treatments, alone or in combination, hoping to find the most effective help for the individual child.

Resources:

Steve Edelson, Ph.D.
Autism Research Institute
4182 Adams Avenue
San Diego, CA 92116
Tel: 1-866-366-3361
www.autism.com (website with extensive information)

Biological Treatments for Autism and PDD, 2nd edition
by William Shaw, Ph.D.
order this and other related books from:
The Great Plains Laboratory Inc.
11813 W. 77th Street
Lenexa, KS 66214
Tel: (913) 341-8949
E-mail: GLP4U@aol.com
www.greatplainslaboratory.com

SPECIAL INTEREST

Clinics in Developmental Medicine No. 126
The Biology of the Autistic Syndromes, 2nd edition
By Christopher Gillberg, M.D. and Mary Coleman, M.D.
1992 Mac Keith Press
Distributed by New York, Cambridge University Press

Kirkman Laboratories
6400 SW Rosewood Street, Lake Oswego, Oregon 97035
Tel: 1-800-245-8282
www.kirkmanlabs.com
(They produce supplements specifically free of casein, gluten, sucrose, artificial colour, flavourings, preservatives, yeast, soy, corn, wheat or milk, as well as vitamin A and D without mercury.)

Autism Network for Dietary Intervention
(provides information and support for using the gluten and casein-free diet)
www.autismndi.com

Samara Blanchard, M.D. (Secretin research)
Associate Professor of Pediatrics
Division of Pediatric Gastroenterology and Nutrition
22 South Greene Street, Box 140/N5W70
Baltimore, MD 21201-1595
Tel: (410) 328-0812
Fax: (410) 328-1072

Jeff Bradstreet, M.D.
International Child Development Resource Center
3800 W. Eau Gallie Blvd., Suite 105, Melbourne, FL 32934
Tel: 321-259-7111
Fax: 321-259-7222
www.icdrc.org/research.html

Amy Holmes, M.D. (Heavy metals)
www.healing-arts.org/children/holmes.htm

Andrew Wakefield, M.D. (MMR vaccine-autism connection research)
Thoughtful House Center for Children
3001 Bee Caves Road, Austin, Texas 78746
Tel: 512 732 8400
Fax: 512 732 8353
www.thoughtfulhouse.org

Jane El-Dahr, M.D. (Immunology)
Department of Pediatrics
Tulane Medical Center
1415 Tulane Ave.
New Orleans, LA 70112
Tel: (504) 588-5800
Fax: (504) 584-3619

http://www.healing-arts.org/children
An extensive informative website overseen and written by:
Lewis E. Mehl-Madrona, MD, PhD
Associate Professor of Family Medicine and Psychiatry
Department of Family Medicine, West Winds Primary Health Centre
University of Saskatchewan College of Medicine
3311 Fairmont Drive, Saskatoon, SK S7M 3Y5, Canada
Tel: 306-655-4249
Fax: 306-655-4894
E-mail: mehlmadrona@aol.com

SPECIAL INTEREST

International Center for
Metabolic Testing
1303 Richmond Rd, Suite 205
Ottawa, ON, CANADA
Tel: (613) 820-6755
Toll free: 1-888-384-7855
Fax: (613) 820-6985
http://www.icmt.com/

Doctor's Data, Inc.
3755 Illinois Avenue, St. Charles, IL
USA 60174-2420
Toll free: 1.800.323.2784
Tel: 1.630.377.8139
Fax: 1.630.587.7860
E-mail: inquiries@doctorsdata.com
www.doctorsdata.com

Metametrix Clinical Laboratory
3425 Corporate Way
Duluth, GA 30096
Tel: 770-446-5483
Toll free: 800-221-4640
www.metametrix.com

Laboratoire Philippe Auguste
119 avenue Philippe Auguste
75011 PARIS, France
Tel: (33) 1.43.72.13.98
Secretary:
Tel: (33) 1.43.67.57.00
Fax: (33) 1.43.79.00.27
E-mail: contact@labbio.net

Other useful websites:
www.autismone.com
www.generationrescue.org
www.generationrescue.org/
    studies.html
www.lymeinducedautism.com

Remember, children are our future.

SPECIAL INTEREST

PREVENTION OF SENSITIZATION TO FOODS IN NEWBORNS AND INFANTS

- Mandatory prenatal counseling for mothers to ensure safe and adequate nutrition during pregnancy.
- In the case of relative infertility, investigate and treat subclinical hypothyroidism.
- Consider conception in the most allergy-free season for both husband and wife (there is an increase of spon- taneous miscarriages in peak seasonal pollination).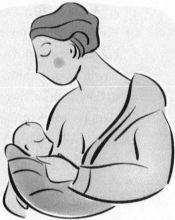
- Do not replace any amalgam fillings before, or during pregnancy, or during breastfeeding.
- Treatment of symptomatic allergies, chemical and food sensitivities with appropriate methods, including desensitization therapy, should be considered.
- Recognition and modification of factors in the nursing mother's diet which cause symptoms.
- **Total breastfeeding, plus occasional water at least to one year of age is highly recommended.**
- Avoid dextrose water, cow's milk or soy formula the in early newborn period, and preferably up until one year if possible.
- Recognize and modify factors in breastfeeding mother's diet that cause symptoms in both mother and infant. Both the mother and infant could be tested with the electrodermal technique.
- Introduce foods singly after age of six months, so that the cause of any symptoms will be easily recognized.
- Introduce foods in a natural, well-cooked, hypoallergenic form.

SPECIAL INTEREST

- Rotate foods after introduction.
- Delay introduction of highly allergenic foods (e.g., grains, cereals, eggs, shellfish, peanuts, and cow's milk) until after one year of age.
- During or after acute viral infections (upper respiratory, gastrointestinal) do not give any new foods and cook familiar ones well.
- Avoid antibiotics during acute illnesses unless a definite bacterial infection is highly probable or has been proven by laboratory testing.
- Use the least medication in the shortest course consistent with adequate care.
- Keep the environment low in allergenic potential; avoid cats, dogs, caged rodents, and horse or stable exposure.
- Provide a bedroom above ground level; avoid bedroom in proximity to downstairs shower, laundry rooms and furnace areas.
- Keep bedroom as dust, mold and chemical-free as possible.
- Avoid painting or renovating.
- No electric blankets or waterbeds.
- Recognize symptoms and try to establish the etiology; treat by the most appropriate methods before illness progresses. Use hypo-sensitization for infants.
- Desensitize for seasonal pollens and symptoms to prevent asthma.
- Provide an absolutely **tobacco- and perfume-free** environment during pregnancy and infancy.
- Simplify foods, i.e., feed single entity foods, not combinations.
- Nutrional supplements or medications can also cause symptoms.

Introduction of Foods by Age

AGE	FOOD	
7 months	Begin with: • peas • squash • carrots • green beans • red beets • sweet potatoes	Then later: • potato • broccoli & cauliflower • cabbage • other peas & beans • other green vegetables • celery, asparagus
8 months	Begin with: • apple (applesauce) • peach • banana	Then later: • apricot • pineapple • plum • cherry • pear • grape
9 months	Begin with: • beef (veal, liver) • pork • lamb	Then later: • fowl (chicken, turkey, duck) • fish • shellfish
10 months	Begin with: • rice • oat • rye	Then later • wheat • millet • barley • corn
1 year	• citrus, eggs, ham, bacon can be introduced • formula or juice should be offered only as a beverage	
After 2 years or later	• nuts, nut butters, seeds • cow's milk	

SPECIAL INTEREST

Juices

Juices should be avoided until one year of age. When used, they should be diluted one part juice to three parts spring water.

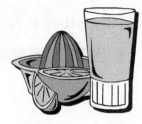

Meats

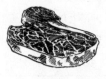

Meats can be offered at around nine months of age, or whenever the baby is ready. This is, of course, after they are tolerating a variety of fruits and vegetables. Processed meats should be avoided.

A Few Rules to Keep in Mind

1. Introduce only one new food per day.
2. **Use organic foods as much as possible.**
3. Do not use tap water; use bottled spring water or filtered tap water.
4. Remember to rotate foods according to the Four-Day Rotation Diet to avoid any sensitivities.
5. Keep a "diet diary," listing the foods given each day and any symptoms observed. It will help you to recognize any food sensitivities that your baby may have.
6. Remember that when foods are cooked, they are less allergic than when eaten raw. Therefore, cooking foods will make them less likely to cause sensitization.

   - If, after the introduction of cow's milk (after the second birthday), your child doesn't like or tolerate it, don't worry; contrary to widespread advertising, it's not vital; adequate calcium can be obtained through other foods and supplements.

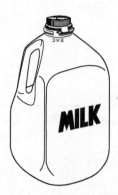

MILK

SPECIAL INTEREST

EPD

Enzyme Potentiated Desensitization (EPD) is a method of immunotherapy developed by Dr. Leonard M. McEwan in England in the mid-60s. It involves desensitization with combinations of a wide variety of very low-dose allergens given with the enzyme beta-glucuronidase, which acts to "potentiate" the immunizing effects of the allergens. EPD is cell-mediated rather than antibody-mediated, resulting in longer-lasting desensitization than any other existing method. EPD is well supported in research

When I first introduced EPD to my practice, I tried it on ten of my "failure" patients—those for whom nothing seemed to work. After several months, 50% had considerable improvement in quality of life, work and function. After ten years of experience with this method, I can say it is one of the most precise, structured, relatively easy, and highly effective treatments available.

It is effective for most individuals and particularly for those who are too fragile to be tested with other methods, and for whom it is difficult to choose medications or supplements due to reactions, or who do not respond well to simple environmental controls and dietary changes.

It is particularly useful for people with severe food sensitivities, chronic asthma, and seasonal allergies. It is very successful in managing children's eczema, learning disabilities, and autism. Success rates reach 80%. It gives the biggest possible umbrella protection for a minimum 220 antigens, including many foods, grasses, trees, weeds, a spectrum of molds, animal danders, bacteria, chemicals. Additional allergens can be used depending on work exposure, e.g., for carpenters, librarians, animal lab workers, etc.

There is a specific and somewhat restrictive dietary and environmental control protocol to be followed for four days around the EPD shot. The stricter the adherence, the better the result. Concomitant therapy with a wide range of supplements before and after the EPD shot improves its effectiveness and corrects nutritional deficiencies. The protocol includes treatment for dysbiosis, from which many patients suffer.

SPECIAL INTEREST

The dose is chosen on an individual basis, i.e., depending on the degree and severity of illness. In the first year, shots are given every two months, in the second year every three months, followed by maintenance with two or three shots per year. Often, after five years, most people can discontinue therapy. When symptoms return, one or two "reminder" shots clear up the problem. Only a few very allergic individuals require longer maintenance. This treatment is well supported scientifically by double-blind studies carried out in Europe, and Dr. McEwen published his research in the Annals of Allergy as early as the 1970s. (See Resources)

HYDROTHERAPY (SAUNA)

In some cases, hydrotherapy may be recommended as part of an individual's treatment for environmental hypersensitivity, and/or for workers intoxicated with solvents, pesticides, etc. Over a period of time, toxins from our food, air and water are deposited and stored in the adipose (fat) tissues of an individual. This buildup of toxins may produce various symptoms and side effects, including increased environmental hypersensitivity. These toxins are slowly released, possibly contributing to the development of chronic degenerative diseases affecting the chest, abdomen, head and extremities. *(Krop J, Chemical Sensitivity After Intoxication at Work with Solvents: Response to Sauna Therapy. The Journal of Alternative and Complementary Medicine, Vol. 4, No. 1, 1998, p. 77-86).*

Hydrotherapy is a detoxification program used to eliminate these toxins from the system. It involves controlled sweating in a sauna under medical supervision, for a prescribed period of time, the calculation of which depends upon the patient's individual tolerance. The therapy also involves taking a prescribed amount of vitamins, minerals, niacin, charcoal and vegetable oil supplements. During the therapy, the amounts of the supplements and blood levels of potassium, sodium, calcium, magnesium and iron are monitored, and measurements of toxic chemicals are taken.

The length of time required for hydrotherapy varies from person to person, depending on the nature and severity of the individual's disease and the individual's tolerance to heat and sweating. Generally, the therapy lasts between three and six weeks and involves four to five individual sessions per week. An intravenous nutrient protocol is recommended two times a week to aid in the detoxification process (see Appendix, p. 327).

SPECIAL INTEREST

HORMONES

HORMONE DISRUPTING CHEMICALS (HDC)

It is imperative to mention the influence of hormone disrupting chemicals globally spread in the environment and their affects on animals and humans. Understandably, it is beyond the scope of this book to describe the issue in detail, nevertheless, a brief outline is helpful. The concept of psycho-nuroimmunoendocrinology was introduced on p. 36.

There is ample evidence available to show how environmental pollutants in our food, water and air adversely affect our central nervous system directly through our olfactory system, causing sensitization of the limbic system; the centre of our emotions. Any minute exposure to solvents, pesticides, and fragrances can cause erratic signaling that in turn can cause not only a change in mood and memory, but also changes in the digestive and respiratory systems and other functions.

There is another mechanism by which man-made toxins spread in the environment and can have a profound effect on the endocrine, central nervous system and the immune system. These chemicals work as hormone disrupters. Reading the book of Theo Colburn, *Our Stolen Future*, published by Penguin Books Canada Ltd., has had a profound influence on me. It re-enforced my long-held observation of the anatomical, behavioural and immune changes in children and adults in my twenty years of practicing environmental medicine.

There are thousands of synthetic chemicals on the market. Each year a thousand new chemicals are developed. In 1989, there were 5 billion pounds of pesticides globally, which includes 1600 chemicals. Now the United States uses thirty times more pesticides than in 1945. In the United States, 2.2 billion pounds of pesticides are used per year, which constitutes 8.8 pounds per capita.

The killing power per pound of pesticides used by 900,000 farms and 69 million households has increased tenfold. Five billion pounds of pesticides are spread globally on agricultural fields, parks, schools, hotels, restaurants, supermarkets, hospitals, nursing homes, homes and gardens. Many of these chemicals have been banned in the United States. In spite of this, in 1991, the United States exported 4.1 million pounds of these banned pesticides,

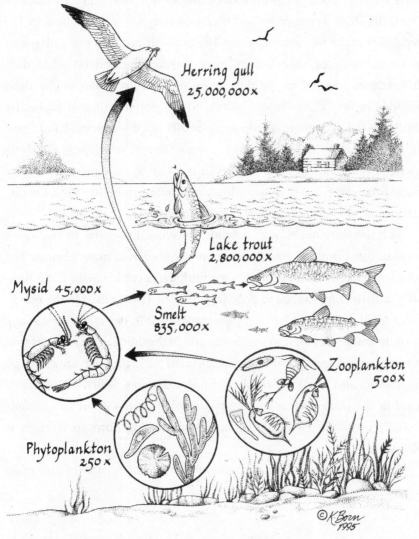

Herring gull
25,000,000×

Lake trout
2,800,000×

Mysid 45,000×

Smelt
835,000×

Zooplankton
500×

Phytoplankton
250×

©K Boon
1995

Our Stolen Future. *Theo Colborn, et al. Penguin Group, 1997.*

including 96 tons of DDT. It is important to remember that we import a variety of foods from these countries, including South America, where banned pesticides are used indiscriminately. These exports also included forty million pounds of pesticides known to be endocrine disrupters.

What Are These Pesticides?

There is a large group of **chlorinated pesticides** with DDT and their metabolites DDE, DDD, as one of the first used massively across the globe since the beginning of the twentieth century. The other chlorinated pesticides, also part of the so-called "Dirty Dozen," include chlordane, lindane, aldrin, dieldrin, endrin, toxifene, heptachlor, mirex, etc. Another group of chemicals included in the "Dirty Dozen" belong to the **polychlorinated biphenyls (PCBs)**, which are composed of a group of 209 possible isomers, 75 different **dioxins**, and 135 **furans**, related to Agent Orange, which was massively sprayed over the jungles and villages in Vietnam by the Americans during the Vietnam War. 2,4-D is also widely and indiscriminately used for cosmetic reasons on our parks, lawns and gardens.

As if this were not enough, scientists recently discovered, to everyone's surprise, that hormone disruptive actions are present in many **plastics**. The active ingredients in many plastics are **phthalates** (which make them flexible); **nonyllphenyl**, added to polyvinyl chloride (PVCs) used in the majority of medical IV equipment, contraceptive creams, detergents, pesticides, the pulp and paper and textile industry, and in the lining of tin cans. **Styrene** is also used in a variety and in vast amounts of packaging, e.g., styrene cups, etc. Plastics also contain **alkylphenol polyetoxylates**, which are manufactured in the United States in amounts ranging from 450 million pounds globally. Another chemical in plastics mimicking hormonal action is **bisphenol-A**.

Additionally, lead, cadmium and mercury are also capable of disrupting hormones.

**What Are The Characteristics of Hormone Disruptor
Chemicals (HDC)?**

- They persist for a long time in the environment; therefore, they are
  also called **persistent chemicals**. For example, the half-life of chlordane is forty years, which means that after forty years, half of the original quantity still persists, not losing its biological activity. In order to
  be classified as a persistent chemical, the substance must have a half-
  life of at least 182 days.

- Their **effect** was observed, **researched** and **proven** on many animals,
  birds, and humans across the globe. Their biological, chemical,
  anatomical, physiological and behavioural effect was observed and
  researched on herring gulls, western gulls, bald eagles, otters, minks,
  alligators, seals, striped dolphins, beluga whales, fish, polar bears,
  laboratory mice and rats, as well as on humans.

- These chemicals **accumulate in animal and human fats.** They are
  easily transported through the placenta. It is interesting that the fetus,
  through the process of bioaccumulation, can store more toxins than
  the mother. These chemicals cross the brain barrier and accumulate in
  the central nervous system. Another mechanism by which animals and
  children absorb these toxins is through breast milk. Breastfed babies
  receive an entire life load of dioxin during the first six months of
  breastfeeding (Steingraber, Sandra *Living Downstream* Addison Wesley,
  1999). There are approximately 250 chemical contaminants in the
  human body, regardless of whether a person lives in China, Russia,
  Eastern or Western Europe, Africa, America or Canada.

- These **hormone-disrupting chemicals are globally distributed** in the
  North and South Pole, the equator, and in all countries. They travel by
  water, air, and food, through migrating birds and fish. They contaminate all species, including human beings, which are at the top of the
  pyramid of the food chain.

- These chemicals, through the process of **bioaccumulation** (particularly PCBs), can increase in level in different species exponentially as they move from animal to animal up the food chain. For example, phytoplankton 250X, zooplankton 500X, lake trout 2,800,000X, and herring gulls 25,000,000X (see illustration p. 271).
- If they act at the very crucial time of the developing embryo, they have a profound effect in extremely **minute amounts**. They act in a fraction of one part per trillion (ppt). To imagine, Theo Colborn tells us to think of one ppt. equaling one drop of gin in 660 train tank cars of tonic water!

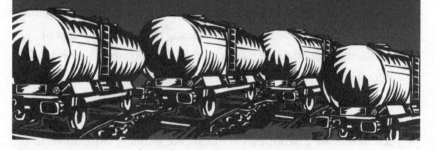

Dose

- **Fraction of one part per trillion (ppt)**
- **10^{-12}**
- **One drop of gin in 660 tank cars filled with tonic water (6 mile long train)**

- These chemicals do not act separately but **act synergistically**. The action of one weak chemical can be potentiated by the presence of others. They can also work through all the mechanisms at the same time. For example, in one organ they can be stimulating, while in another they could be blocking.

SPECIAL INTEREST

- Persistent chemicals do not work like other toxins in the linear fashion, as is our understanding of toxicology; i.e., bigger dose—higher response. **They act in a non-linear fashion**. It means, as has been proven in animals, that smaller doses are more potent and effective and produce more profound effects, particularly if they act in the specific vulnerable time of the developing embryo.
- It is interesting to note that persistent chemicals not only have a general toxic effect in laboratory animals and humans, but also affect offspring up to the second and third generation. The changes noted in offspring are not seen in mothers.

What Is Their Mechanism of Action?

- Physiologically, hormones have regulatory influences on all tissues and organs. Persistent chemicals affect the endocrine system by mimicking the actions of the hormones. Hormone disruptors acting on embryos and the developing fetus create anatomical changes in the urinary and genital organs of both males and females. They cause malfunctions in behavioural and sexual orientation, affect immune functions and, through their effect on the thyroid, cause central nervous system problems up to the third generation.
- Chemical structures of these substances resemble the **steroid hormones**, both female (estrogen, progesterone) and male (testosterone), the **adrenal hormones** (cortisol), as well as the **thyroid hormones**. Because of their similarities, they can mimic the action of estrogen (estrogen mimickers, xenoestrogens). They can also block the receptors for the normally occurring physiological action of hormones. Sex, adrenal and thyroid hormones have a profound effect on the development of psychological characteristics and sexual behaviour of both males and females through their action on the central nervous system.

- There is a specific **window of time** during the development of the embryo of an animal or human when any disturbance of the regular physiological process leads to catastrophic consequences for the developing fetus, resulting in the physical and anatomical disruption of the sex organs of children, as well as psychological deviations in sexual orientation in later life. These chemicals, particularly PCBs, also affect the thyroid hormones through the blocking of the receptors of normal thyroid hormones. By doing so, they affect the developing brain, and children are born with low IQ's, overactive or violent behaviour, and with learning disabilities.

So What Are The Observable Changes in Animals and Humans?

- Before seven weeks, the developing embryo that has either XX (female) or XY (male) genetic material, is unisex with two different tissue systems. The Wolffian and Mullerian ducts develop either into a penis or scrotum and testicles (Wolffian tissue), or, in the case of a female, the clitoris, labia and vagina (Mullerian tissue). This window of time in the development of the embryo is after seven weeks into the pregnancy, when the sex is determined, i.e., the appropriate gene on either the XY or XX chromosome will signal the unisex glands to develop into either male or female. If the hormone-disrupting chemicals are present at that time, the development is altered and the changes are observable in the child's or adult's life.

  If estrogen-mimicking chemicals interfere, we observe in boys an underdeveloped penis, undescended testicles (they may remain in the inguinal canal or abdomen), cysts in the epididymis, (the place for maturing sperm), underdeveloped testicles and a higher rate of cancer of the testicles and prostate.

We are already witnessing a drop in the number of sperm from 116 to 128 million per ml to fifty to sixty million per ml of ejaculate from 1940 to 1990. This study was done by Danish scientist Niels Skakkeback and was published in the *British Journal of Medicine* in 1992. Other researchers observed not only small volumes of sperm, but also anatomical abnormalities (double-headed or double-tailed sperm), loss of mobility and increase of viscosity, all leading to lower fertility.

The same mimicking estrogen in girls can produce an enlarged clitoris, an abnormal shape of the vagina or uterus, and premature puberty. In later life, ectopic pregnancies, miscarriages, premature babies, endometriosis, obesity, osteoporosis and an increased rate of cancer of the breast, ovaries and uterus may occur. These abnormalities definitely interfere with the fertility and reproduction process of the human and animal species.

Additionally, both boys and girls may have anatomical abnormalities in the urinary tract, e.g., hypospadiasis (opening of the urethra on the underside of the penis instead of at the tip), a short or double urethra, a single, double or abnormal kidney. These hormone-disrupting chemicals are also able to change the sexual orientation in the development stage.

The most extreme example of what could happen when something blocks the hormonal message is a **feminizing male**, who has the XY chromosomes of a male, testicles in the abdomen (undescended) and tissues unresponsive to testosterone. This person looks and behaves like a female but does not menstruate. They never develop the body, brain or sexual behaviour of a male in spite of the genetic and chromosomal material.

- **Vinclozolin**, a chemical widely used to kill fruit fungus as well as DDE, a metabolite of DDT, works as an androgen blocker, which will derail boys' sexual development, resulting in different forms of "intersex" or hermaphrodite characteristics.

- These persistent chemicals also have an affect on brain development and behaviour. Female rats, mice, hamsters and guinea pigs, if exposed to estrogenic chemicals, show more masculinization and decreased feminization characteristics of behaviour. In different studies, a considerable percentage of daughters whose mothers were treated with **DES (diethylstilbestrol)**, a drug used extensively on many women during 1950 to 1980, reported life-long bisexual and homo- sexual orientation. Both sons and daughters of those exposed mothers experienced an increased rate of anxiety, anorexia nervosa, phobias, neurosis, and major depressive states.

- Another large class of fungicide are members of the **piridine carbinol family**, as well as DDE. These chemicals could interfere with the cholesterol metabolism, causing a generalized depletion of all hormones derived from cholesterol: adrenal hormones (cortisol), and gonadal hormones (testosterone, estrogen and progesterone).

- **PCBs, along with their isomers,** and **dioxins** have a negative effect on the brain, hypothalmus, pituitary gland and other hormonal glands. They interfere with and block thyroid hormone receptors that are responsible for brain development. It is estimated that approximately 5% of children suffering from **hyperactivity and learning disabilities** have been exposed to PCBs and dioxin in utero. Both animals and children exposed to hormone disruptors in the womb show behavioural problems, aggression, and low resistance to stress (physical, chemical and psychological). These children show poor behaviour, and a decrease in intelligence and capacity for social organization. Altered action of thyroid hormones and/or low levels of adrenal hormones (cortisol is known as a stress-protective hormone), as well as altered immunity, can lead to what we see in general practice: chronic fatigue syndrome, general inability to cope with stress, increased infections and a massive increase in autoimmune diseases, such as Hashimoto Thyroiditis, Graves disease, rheumatoid arthritis, lupus, and cardiovas- cular disease.

- It is proven that persistent chemicals can lower the number of T-helper cells and T-suppressor cells, leading to increases in viral infections, AIDS, bacterial and fungal infections (e.g., candida), as well as the explosion of allergic disorders and chemical sensitivities seen in the practices of environmental medicine.

> WE HAVE TO REMEMBER THAT THE FUNDAMENTAL REGULATION OF THE DEVELOPMENT OF ALL SPECIES, WHETHER IT BE MICE, BATS, OTTERS, SEALS, DEER, ALLIGATORS, WHALES, OR HUMANS, DEPENDS ON THE SAME HORMONES, AND IN THE END, ALL SPECIES, INCLUDING HUMANS, SHARE THE SAME FATE.
>
> WHAT IS ASTONISHINGLY DISTURBING IS THE FACT THAT WE AS HUMANS, WHETHER POORLY OR HIGHLY EDUCATED, CONTINUE TO USE THESE CHEMICALS IN OUR DAILY LIVES WITHOUT THINKING OF THE CONSEQUENCES.

THE MOST COMMON HORMONAL PROBLEMS

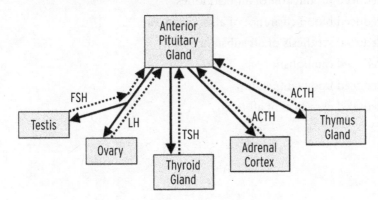

SPECIAL INTEREST

All stimulating hormones (FSH, LH, TSH, etc.) are secreted by the anterior pituitary gland, sending signals to the peripheral glands, the testes, ovaries, thyroid gland, adrenal cortex and the thymus gland. The peripheral glands send signals back to the pituitary gland, resulting in a self-regulating mechanism. All functions are very closely related.

THYROID GLAND

The thyroid gland, sometimes called the "forgotten gland," is responsible for the control of the entire body's metabolism. Such things as energy and growth, heat regulation, blood circulation, immune function and removal of waste products all fall under the supervision of the thyroid gland.

The prime hormone is T3 (triiodothyronine), which works on the level of every tissue in the body. T3 is enzymatically converted from T4 (tetra-iodothyronine), which is dependent on selenium, iron, cortisol, zinc, B12, folic acid and B2.

Thyroid diseases, particularly the autoimmune disorder Hashimoto's thyroiditis, have increased dramatically, due in part to exposure to nuclear radiation (see page 311).

Too much thyroid hormone is called hyperthyroidism, and too little hormone is called hypothyroidism, which is more common.
Resultant effects of hypothyroidism:

- Reduced production of all hormones
- Reduced blood clearance of all substances
- Reduced synthesis of all substances
- Reduced catabolism
- Reduced body temperature
- Reduced excretion of all toxins

SPECIAL INTEREST

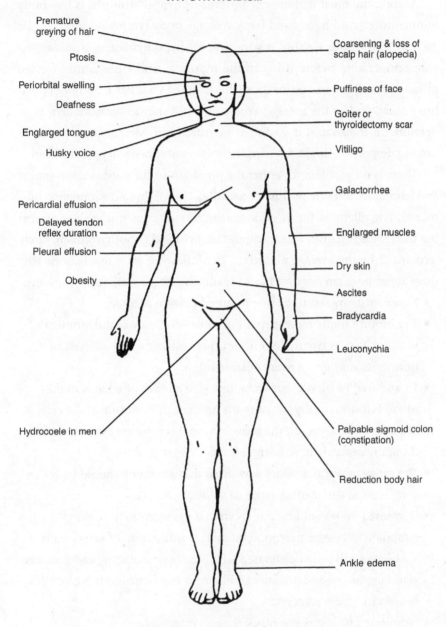

HYPOTHYROIDISM

Premature greying of hair

Ptosis

Periorbital swelling

Deafness

Englarged tongue

Husky voice

Pericardial effusion

Delayed tendon reflex duration

Pleural effusion

Obesity

Hydrocoele in men

Coarsening & loss of scalp hair (alopecia)

Puffiness of face

Goiter or thyroidectomy scar

Vitiligo

Galactorrhea

Englarged muscles

Dry skin

Ascites

Bradycardia

Leuconychia

Palpable sigmoid colon (constipation)

Reduction body hair

Ankle edema

Schematic Illustration of Symptoms Associated with Hypothyroidism

Among the most irritating symptoms of hypothyroidism is low body temperature (cold hands and feet). Average body temperature should be 36.6 to 36.8 degree Celsius. A good test for hypothyroidism is measuring your temperature before rising in the morning, under the armpit for ten minutes over five consecutive days (this is called your Basal Body Temperature) and calculate the average. Women should start to measure their temperature on the second day of their menstruation. Mental sluggishness to varying degrees or "brain fog" are also experienced with hypothyroidism.

There is no problem for either the physician or the patient if symptoms and laboratory tests are positive (a sensitive TSH or thyroid stimulating hormone). The dilemma for most doctors occurs when symptoms are present but the TSH is negative. This is so-called **subclinical hypothyroidism**, rarely recognized by the average physician. The following are a few reasons why there are quite often negative blood results but positive clinical symptoms:

- Never trust any test to be one hundred percent accurate.
- The blood sample represents a hormone level only at the moment of venipuncture. A twenty-four hour urine collection and analysis of hormones may give a more reliable result.
- T3 and free T4 blood tests sometime give an idea of what is in the blood but don't really measure the amount of hormone in the cells.
- Research volunteers, on the basis of whom norms are established, do not necessarily have normal levels.
- The range of normal values is wide so that any value should be compared to the median range of values.
- Decreased blood volume due to arterial vasoconstriction, slow lymphatic drainage, mucopolysaccharide infiltration of vessel walls.
- TSH levels will only be elevated when the hypothalamus and pituitary gland are not myxedematous and thyroid hormone levels are very low as seen in advanced cases.
- Hormone disruptors can block the cell receptors.

Therefore, **if** there are:
- Clinical signs and symptoms
- Familial history
- Positive results with Basal Body Temperature test
- Positive thyroid antibody
- But normal TSH,

then:
- A **therapeutic trial** should be implemented and if there is a positive response to the therapy, then this is an indication for therapy to be continued.

Choice of Therapy

The great majority of medical doctors use the synthetic thyroid L-thyroxine or levothyroxine (T4), with such product trade names as Eltroxin or Synthroid. Unfortunately, T4 is only a precursor and, in order to be biologically active it has to be metabolized to T3 (triiodothyronine), which is the real metabolically active hormone utilized by all tissues.

Since the hypothyroid state creates poor, slow metabolism, the conversion of T4 to T3 is slow or inadequate, and the final result is that the amount of T3 delivered to the cells is poor. Using T4, the TSH can be normalized, but the patient still has a lot of symptoms of hypothyroidism: Use of natural thyroid that contains a mixture of T3 and T4, or use of T3 alone, is preferable and gives better clinical results. T3 acts on cell membranes, facilitating the entry of amino acids and sugars; on mitochondria to synthesize ATP, the major substance responsible for appropriate energy; and on the cell nucleus receptor for gene expression.

Sometimes it could be sufficient to give a homeopathic remedy such as Thyroidea, which can substantially help the subclinically malfunctioning thyroid. An appropriate dose could be evaluated with the help of any electrodermal equipment, as well as blood tests and clinical symptoms.

SPECIAL INTEREST

It may take time to find a doctor who understands these subtle differences and who will treat subclinical hypothyroidism.

The proper function of the thyroid gland, and secretion of the appropriate amount of hormones, depend particularly on nutrients such as selenium, iron, vitamins B1, B2, B12 and folic acid. Supplementation with these important vitamins and minerals is essential.

Hyperthyroidism is the opposite of hypothyroidism. Although it is much easier to diagnose, treatment is more difficult, requiring the expertise of an endocrinologist.

ADRENAL GLAND

The adrenal glands are small glands located on top of the kidneys. The function of the adrenal glands and their respective hormones include:

- Resistance to both mental and physical stress
- Maintenance of energy
- Protection against hypoglycemia (low blood sugar)
- Maintaining electrolyte balance between potassium and sodium
- Maintaining normal blood pressure—this is the action of aldosterone
- Androgenic effect (DHEA, androstenol): maintain the growth and repair of tissue after injury
- Estrogenic effect: protection against hot flashes during normal menses and production of estrogen (postmenopausal)
- Development and maintenance of normal immunity

Adrenal hormones are very closely related to the function of the thyroid gland. A number of different hormones are secreted from the adrenal glands. These hormones are essential for life.

Patients with subclinically low adrenal function present with a number of **complaints and symptoms**:

- Excessive fatigue
- Nervousness and irritability, apprehension

- Depression
- Generalized weakness
- Lightheadedness, fainting spells
- Insomnia
- Inability to concentrate, confusion
- Poor memory
- Frustration
- Headache
- Heart palpitations
- Craving for salt and/or sweets
- Alcohol intolerance, food and drug intolerance
- Anorexia
- Premenstrual tension
- Neck and shoulder pain

On examination, the patient may present with the following:
- Postural hypotension (dizziness or blacking out after standing up from a supine position)
- Recurrent inflammation of cervical (neck) vertebrae
- Thin and dry skin
- Poor perspiration
- Thinning hair
- Low blood pressure

Mild or subclinical **adrenal insufficiency** may occur in:
- Chronic stress
- Post viral syndrome (influenza, mononucleosis, Epstein Barr virus, hepatitis)
- Chronic allergic disorders (rhinitis, asthma)
- Autoimmune disorders such as rheumatoid arthritis, diabetes mellitus, chronic thyroiditis

SPECIAL INTEREST

Appropriate lab tests can help to diagnose these conditions by finding the following markers:

- The level of cortisol measured before and after stimulation with ACTH (adrenocorticotrophic hormone)
- Elevated eosinophil levels (type of white blood cell) in the blood
- Flat glucose tolerance curve (hypoglycemic curve)
- Low 17-ketosteroids (hormones secreted by adrenals)
- 24-hour urine collection for cortisol

Treatment may include removal of the primary cause of the problem (e.g., recurrent infections, allergies, chronic stress). The most successful treatment is with a physiological dose of cortisone (5mg) four times a day with small meals. Steroids (cortisone is a steroid hormone) have an unfortunate reputation. There is general public resistance against the use of this hormone. However, there is a difference between a physiological dose and a pharmacological dose, as in the use of asthma. A physiological dose of 5mg four times a day is safe and does not produce any side effects and, in fact, can help tremendously (Jeffries, W. Safe Uses of Cortisone. Chas. Thomas 1981).

Some physicians use adrenal extracts of animal origin. Licorice root, Vitamin C, and pantothenic acid are also capable of naturally stimulating cortisol production. In mild cases, use of homeopathic remedies such as glandula supranulis by injection or sublingual route can be very effective.

Anytime a pharmacological dose of steroid, e.g., prednisone, is used for asthma, nephrotic syndrome, or lupus, etc., then protection of the adrenal glands should be considered with such measures as concomitant use of DHEA.

PREMENSTRUAL SYNDROME (PMS)

- PMS affects approximately 45% of women and has a negative impact on their lives. This is a cluster of physical and psychological symptoms, which occur either around ovulation on the 12th to 14th day, or just before menstrual flow.

Physical symptoms include:

bloating	diarrhea or constipation
weight gain	breast swelling and/or tenderness
swelling	headache
acne	joint or muscle pain
nausea	clumsiness, poor coordination
shaking	dizziness
insomnia	hot and cold feelings
seizures	

Emotional symptoms include:

restlessness	sugar and/or salt cravings
mood swings	increased appetite
anxiety	irritability
confusion	suicidal thoughts
forgetfulness	unexplained crying spells, etc.

What can you do? Even though a single cause of PMS is not known, it seems to be that a correction of environmental and dietary conditions plays a large role in helping this condition. Below is a list of recommendations to improve PMS symptoms:

- Elimination of sensitive foods (most often sugar, wheat, alcohol, yeast, coffee, etc.)
- Assessing and correcting thyroid and adrenal functions
- Treating any underlying infections (e.g., yeast)
- Supplements: 50 to 200mg of vitamin B6 per day and other B-complex vitamins, 400 to 700mg of magnesium per day and other minerals (e.g., zinc and chromium), 400 to 800I.U. of vitamin E per day, and essential oils (evening primrose and flax)
- Desensitization of progesterone and/or estrogen by SDEPT provocation and neutralization method

SPECIAL INTEREST

- Use of natural progesterone cream or capsules prepared by a compounding pharmacy
- L-tryptophan, 500mg taken three times a day
- Neutralization for neurotransmittors such as serotonin, dopamine, and histamine
- Use of potassium iodine, and preferably aqueous diatomic iodine, is very effective in treating breast pain and swelling
- If all these natural methods fail, then pharmaceutical methods may be useful such as antiprostaglandins, diuretics, and antidepressants. Recently, in some psychiatric circles, PMS has been considered to be primarily a psychiatric disorder and treated with antidepressants such as Prozac, an insult to millions of women!

MENOPAUSE IS NOT A DISEASE

Menopause is the time in the life of a woman when menstrual functions cease. This happens at approximately 50 years of age. The body prepares for this event during a period called "perimenopause," which lasts for about ten years from forty to fifty years of age. Symptoms begin which reflect the diminishing function of the ovaries. At this time, there is not only a progressive decline in hormonal function of the ovaries, but also a lack of balance among estrogen, progesterone and androgen (testosterone) levels. Perimenopause begins with symptoms of progesterone deficiency and ends with estrogen deficiency. Symptoms of androgen deficiency should also be evaluated.

The table below lists symptoms due to the lack of the three important hormones. Note how many symptoms are related to the central nervous system. This hormonal deficiency is often misinterpreted and treated with antidepressants instead of balancing the hormone levels.

SYMPTOMS:	Knowledge of symptoms permits assessment of an adequate E_2-P-A Balance	
HORMONE DEFICIENCY	PHYSICAL	CNS RELATED
Lack of Progesterone (P)	• Painful, swollen breasts • Swelling • Excessive menstruation • Water retention • Constant abdominal pain at menstruation	• Excessive nervousness • Anxiety, irritability • Insomnia
Lack of Estrogen (E_2)	• Dry mucous membranes, especially vaginal • Wrinkles • Poor or no menstruation • Painful menstrual cramps	• Constant tiredness • Depression • Libido lessening
Lack of Androgen (A)	• Muscular hypotrophy • Wrinkles • Muscular weakness	• Loss of sense of dominance • Loss of self-confidence • Loss of libido

There are a number of factors which may affect the function of hormones at any time in the life of an individual, but in the perimenopausal phase, any disturbance of these functions is particularly annoying. The aim of the practitioner is not only to prescribe appropriate (natural) hormones but also to correct any negative factors which may affect hormonal function:

Adequate diet

- Decrease excessive caloric intake
- Increase fibre consumption
- Decrease excessive protein intake

SPECIAL INTEREST

- Decrease fat consumption (saturated fats, transfatty acids, e.g., fried foods)
- Take appropriate vitamin and mineral supplementation

Adequate life style

- Sunlight
- Adequate sleep
- Exercise
- Normal/balanced stress
- Adequate emotional expression
- Spirituality

Avoidance of environmental toxins

- Coffee, alcohol, tobacco, margarine, anticancer drugs, tranquilizers, antidepressants, anesthetics, some antifungal drugs, antiparkinson and antiparasitic drugs, narcotics, heavy metals (mercury, lead and cadmium), all insecticides and herbicides, food additives, industrial chemicals, plastics, solvents, etc. (see Hormone Disrupting Chemicals, page 270).

Avoidance of

- Hysterectomy and tubal ligation (both result in disturbance of blood supply and atrophy)

When replacement therapy is indicated, the goal is to use natural hormones. These are pharmacologically modified substances usually derived from wild yams, soy or clover. The best-known products are: estriol, progesterone, and dehydroepiandrosterone (DHEA). There is a difference in the metabolic action between natural and synthetic hormones. Natural hormones are more easily metabolized and are biodegradable in the environment and there are no harmful side effects.

The following are side effects of synthetic hormones:

SYNTHETIC ESTROGEN E.G., PREMARIN	SYNTHETIC PROGESTERONE E.G., PROVERA
• Derived from pregnant mare's urine	• Lowers HDL (good cholesterol)
• Difficult to metabolize, accumulates in the liver	• Increases angiotensin and rennin (causes hypertension)
• A xenoestrogen in the environment	• Causes hirsutism (excessive hair growth on face and extremities)
• Increases blood pressure	
• Increases thrombogenic effect (vein and artery thrombosis)	
• Increases risk of uterine fibromas	
• Increases risk of breast and uterine cancer	

Synthetic androgen, because of its ability to increase muscle strength, is often used illegally by athletes. There are some herbs that exhibit hormonal activity and these are often used to successfully treat menopausal symptoms. They include:

- Dong Quai (angelica sinensis), widely used for menopausal symptoms
- Tribulus terrestris is used for hot flashes, insomnia, depression, loss of libido
- Chaste berry, which can increase progesterone and decrease estrogen
- Black cohosh, useful in menopausal depression

Careful and thoughtful hormonal replacement with natural hormones can:
- **Increase the quality of life** (dynamism, cheerfulness, self-confidence, sexual drive)
- **Decrease aging symptoms** (wrinkles, thinning of skin, muscle flabbiness, spine degeneration, hirsutism, uterine and bladder prolapse)
- **Decrease or reverse aging pathologies** such as osteoporosis, atherosclerosis, cardiovascular disease, breast cysts, uterine fibromas, ovarian cysts
- **Prevent** cancer of the breast, uterus, and ovaries
- **Increase survival rate**

SPECIAL INTEREST

STEALTH INFECTIONS

The "germ theory" dominated the late nine-
teenth and early twentieth centuries. In over
thirty years of medical practice, I, as well as
many other physicians, have noted a shift
from a predominance of acute infections to a
predominance of more chronic and degenerative diseases. Does this mean that infections
no longer play an important role in our life,
or is it that they play a role not recognized in
degenerative disease? What are the factors
contributing to this switch in the manifestation of diseases?

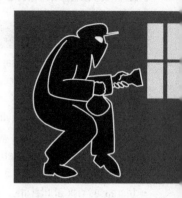

There is definitely a profound influence by our polluted environment
and climate change on all species, including humans and microbial organisms (bacteria, fungi, viruses, parasites). Under these circumstances, all
species undergo accelerated evolutionary changes.

Pollutants affect the individual (host) on a low-level basis (low dose,
big effect). Toxic pollutants decrease beneficial soil organisms, creating an
imbalance in favour of pathological species. Additionally, toxins penetrate
the human species through food changes (pesticides, antibiotics, chlorine,
massive use of pharmaceuticals) and not only deplete the friendly, protective
bacteria in our gut, but also act as immunosuppressors, disturbing hormones and neurotransmitters (the endocrine, immune, and nervous systems are the three pillars of homeostasis).

Acid rain, industries, toxins, pharmaceuticals, poor and dangerous farming methods, food processing, transportation and lengthy storage of food,
an increase of heavy metals in soil, air, and water, all decrease the nutrient content in our foods. This, in turn, disturbs our metabolism and
puts our genetic code into shock, which then tries to repair and build cells
from deficient raw materials (nutrients), in turn creating weaker and more
vulnerable future generations.

There is an ever increasing number of people living in an unnatural environment enclosed in steel, glass, cement, plastic, and ever surrounded by increasing electromagnetic fields emanating from modern gadgets. In this environment, we also live with "domesticated" cats and dogs, meaning they are different from their wild ancestors through genetic manipulations thanks to human influence and breeding. Virtually all the plants and animals we eat today (unless certified as "organic") are genetically modified. In addition, the media bombards us with often negative and conflicting news.

This causes destabilization in our mental and physical health, decreases our vigilance to protect ourselves from microorganisms, which also undergo evolutionary changes and become more insidiously sophisticated (remember, we are their prey) for their survival and multiplication.

There is growing scientific evidence that most of the degenerative diseases of our modern times are caused by microorganisms. The reason this connection is not recognized is the minimal funding for development and research into appropriate tests for detection. There is also a lack of a distinct acute phase at the beginning of the infectious process as seen in all infections of the ninteenth and beginning of the twentieth centuries, when signs and symptoms were obvious to the suffering and easily recognized by MDs.

Most of the human diseases that were accepted as infectious during the last twenty-five years have actually been chronic. They have been referred to as "stealth" infections. The scientific debate continues as to whether the presence of pathogens found in the lesions of chronic degenerative diseases are causative factors or just bystanders. Nevertheless, careful use of some antimicrobial agents in some degenerative diseases such as rheumatoid arthritis (RA) or scleroderma can bring a very pleasant surprise both to the physician and, especially, the suffering patient.

Following are examples of the relationship between chronic diseases and existing pathogens:

SPECIAL INTEREST

DISEASE	PATHOGENS
Atherosclerotic heart disease Multiple sclerosis Alzheimer's disease	Chlamydia pneumoniae – in acute phases causes pneumonia
Ulcers of stomach and duodenum	Helicobacter pylori
Schizophrenia	Toxoplasma gondi infecting rodents but transmitted by cats to humans
Juvenile obsessive compulsive disorder	Streptococcal infections
Collagen diseases (rheumatoid arthritis, scleroderma, etc.)	Mycoplasmas
Chronic fatigue syndrome (CFS) Bipolar depression Schizophrenia	Borna virus affecting horses, sheep, cats, rodents
Cervical cancer	Human papillovirus
Liver cancer	Hepatitis C virus
CFS	Human herpes virus (HHV-6)
Multiple myeloma	Human herpes virus (HHV-8)
Dandruff, acne, warts, halitosis, athlete's foot, gingivitis	Caused by infections

There is also an association between stealth viruses and Lyme disease: they attack the cells of the host, creating a favourable environment for the growth of intracellular bacteria such as Borrelia burgdorferi, ehrlichia and babesia, the causative agents for chronic and devastating Lyme disease.

It is difficult to detect these pathogens, which penetrate cells deeply, as there is no one technique that may diagnose this problem. Awareness of these pathogens, a good clinical history and a combination of specialized laboratory tests are required before a trial of therapy.

Knowing about stealth infections gives a new perspective in helping many patients with chronic degenerative disease using the precepts of Environmental Medicine, careful and appropriate selection of different antimicrobial agents, protecting the gut with probiotics, as well as supporting the immune system with a variety of immune stimulants. For instance, Dr. V. Thomas McPherson Brown's Protocol for collagen diseases is very helpful.

Resources:

Center for Complex Infectious Diseases
3328 Stevens Avenue
Rosemead, CA 91770
www.ccid.org

Bowen Research and Training Institute Incorporated
Lake Alfred
245 North Seminole Avenue,
Lake Alfred, Florida 33850
Tel: 863.956.3538
www.bowen.org

DENTAL AMALGAMS

To replace or not to replace, is another serious controversy in medical science and politics today. According to Health Canada guidelines (not enforceable) of August 1996, dentists should not put any mercury amalgams into children up to eighteen years of age, pregnant women, anyone receiving steroid therapy or having kidney problems. Dentists were ordered to place removed amalgams into hazardous waste containers because amalgam has a highly toxic effect on the environment and fish particularly. Apparently it's safe for everyone else—strange logic!

Countries such as Sweden, Germany and other Scandinavian countries have totally or partially banned the use of silver amalgam fillings. In Canada, a class action suit against the Dental College, Health Canada, and mercury manufacturers was started in August 1996 by some dentists and citizens (**www.talkinternational.com/mercury.htm**).

There are different forms of mercury which all have a toxic effect:
- Elemental: quicksilver (vapourizes—used in dental amalgams)
- Inorganic: mercuric and mercurous salts (Hg+1, Hg+2—used as antiseptic)
- Organic: ethyl, dimethyl, etc. (merthiolate or thimerosal—used as preservatives in vaccines)

According to the World Health Organization, common sources of mercury intoxication in micrograms of mercury absorbed per day are:
- Dental amalgams   – 3.0 to 17.0
- Fish/seafood   – 2.34
- Water   – 0.0035
- Air   – 0.001

If we all agree that mercury is a highly toxic poison, then Dr. Huggins of Colorado, one of the pioneers in recognizing mercury amalgam problems, must be right (*It's All in Your Head, Diseases Caused by Silver Mercury Amalgam Fillings*, Huggins, H.A. and Huggins S.A., Avery Press, 1993).

Mercury is stored in the kidneys, liver, heart, all neurological tissues, and endocrine organs.

Factors such as acidic foods, chewing, teeth grinding, number and filling size, all increase the release of mercury into the body. Another factor is buccal galvanic current (electricity generated in the mouth); particularly dangerous are gold crowns covering amalgam fillings or located beside teeth with amalgam fillings. Even more dangerous are root canals, which become a source of hidden infections that produce toxins such as hydrogen sulphite (H_2S) or methylthiol, which binds to mercury, producing methyl mercury compounds—very dangerous and toxic substances. These toxins have an affinity to fats and lipids, particularly in the central nervous system

There is ample anecdotal evidence that some long-lasting debilitating symptoms have disappeared dramatically and quickly in many patients after removal of amalgam fillings. To my own surprise, I saw this in my own environmental medical practice. This immediate improvement often takes place where high buccal galvanic current interrupting nerve conductions was cleared by removing amalgams or metal crowns.

In general, I believe that no one should have amalgam fillings, but the decision to have them removed has to be carefully balanced. On the one hand, you have the monetary cost and possible complications such as losing teeth or ending up with a root canal; and on the other hand, you have the improved health benefits of mercury removal.

SPECIAL INTEREST

Dental amalgams can cause many symptoms:

AFFECTED BODY SYSTEM	MERCURY SYMPTOM
Cardiovascular System	Angina, heart attack, heart murmur, irregular heart beat, pressure in chest, tachycardia, unexplained chest pains
Central Nervous System	Convulsions, chronic headache, dizziness, dim vision, difficulties walking, epilepsy, facial twitching, failure of muscle coordination, insomnia, hearing difficulties, loss of ability to perform movement of the hands, mental disability, muscle paralysis, muscle twitching, multiple sclerosis, noises or sounds in the head, narrowing of field of vision, numbness of arms and legs, ringing in the ears, speech disorders, tremor of hands, feet and lips, tingling of fingers and toes, tingling of lips and nose, unexplained leg jerks
Digestive System	Colitis, constipation, diarrhea, digestive problems, diverticulitis, frequent bloating, frequent heartburn, loss of appetite, nausea, stomach cramps, ulcers
Endocrine System	Adrenal dysfunction, chronic low body temperature, cold hands and feet, diabetes, diabetic tendency, edema, frequent urination especially at night, hypo-glycemia, ovary dysfunction, prostate problems, thyroid dysfunction, weight loss
Energy Levels	Chronic fatigue, drowsiness, irregular breathing, lack of energy, lethargy, muscle weakness, oversleeping, tiredness
Immune System	Allergies, asthma, cancer, chronic fatigue, environmental illness, Epstein-Barr virus, Hodgkin's disease, immune deficiency disease, leukemia, mononucleosis, rhinitis, sinusitis, susceptibility to flu, colds, etc., swollen glands

SPECIAL INTEREST

Oral Cavity	Bad breath, bleeding gums, bone loss around teeth, burning sensation in mouth, enlarged salivary glands, increased flow of saliva, leukoplakia, loosening of teeth, loss of teeth, metallic taste in mouth, mouth ulcers, periodontal (gum) disease, purple-black pigment in gums, sore throat, persistent cough, stomatitis, swollen tongue and glands, tendency towards tartar formation
Psychological & Behavioral	Anxiety, apathy, confusion and depression, difficulty making decisions, emotional instability, fits of anger, forgetfulness, hallucinations, inability to concentrate, irritability, lack of self-control, lowered intelligence, manic-depression, nervousness, nightmares, psychological disturbances, short attention span, short-term memory loss, sleep disturbances, tension, unexplained suicidal ideas
Skin	Acne, dermatitis, excessive itching, rashes (eczema patches), rough skin, skin flushes
Others	Anemia, arthritis, birth defects in offspring, candida albicans (persistent), joint pains, kidney stones, leg cramps, nephritis or symptoms of kidney disease, slow healing

SPECIAL INTEREST

When removing amalgams, the following should be considered:
- All patients, and especially chemically sensitive ones, should be tested for compatibility to various composite materials which will be used as a replacement for amalgams.
- Replacement should be done by a dentist trained in biological dentistry.
- Removal of amalgams must be accomplished with adequate protection from mercury vapour (rubber dam, oxygen mask, air filtration, etc.).

See *Nutritional Supplement Protocol for Dental Amalgam Replacement* in the
Appendix

Each tooth is connected through energy meridians to a major organ in the
body. Therefore, any acute or chronic dental infection (root canals, cavita-
tions, gum disease) or buccal current (an electrical current produced by the
metal amalgam) has enormous influence on the general state of health.
Considering the impact of dental probems on health, denticare could be as
useful as, or more useful than, medicare in its present form.

FOR MORE INFORMATION ON MERCURY AMALGAMS: INTER-
NATIONAL ACADEMY OF ORAL MEDICINE AND TOXICOLOGY
CHAMPIONS GATE, FL, (863) 420-6373: WWW.IAOMT.ORG.
OTHER WEBSITES: WWW.ALTCORP.COM, WWW.GOOGLE.COM/
TOP/HEALTH/ALTERNATIVE/NON-TOXIC_LIVING/
MERCURY_AND_AMALGAMS/. VIDEO SHOWING HOW MERCURY
DESTROYS NEURONS: HTTP://APOLLO.UCALGARY.CA/MERCURY/
MOVIES.

SPECIAL INTEREST

CANCER

CAUSES AND PREVENTION

This topic is broad, complicated and inexhaustible. Hundreds of books and thousands of scientific papers are published on this issue. Nevertheless, some common sense and practical approaches to this issue deserve mention in this guide.

Cancer is the second leading cause of death in North America, after cardiovascular disease. The dramatic increase in the last forty years represents an epidemic. Within the next twenty years, one-third of our population will get some form of cancer in their lifetime, and one-quarter will die from it.

An increase in the incidence of cancer from 1950 to 1990, age adjusted, is as follows:

- Breast cancer, estrogen-receptor positive—135%
- Prostate and testicular cancer—100% each
- Multiple myeloma, non-Hodgkin's lymphoma—200%
- Childhood cancers—greater than 200%
- Brain and nervous system cancers—40%
- In the age group of 28–35 years, the cancer rate has gone up 300%.

We must consider the possibility that the increase in cancer has something to do with the quantity of chemicals polluting our environment. In 1940, we produced one billion pounds of new synthetic chemicals. By 1950, this had increased to fifty billion pounds. The majority of these chemicals include a broad range of neurotoxic, endocrinotoxic, immunotoxic and carcinogenic substances. Since 1950, thousands more chemicals have been added to the environment. Presently two thousand new chemicals are introduced annually.

In Canada, Saskatchewan has the highest rate of breast and cervical cancer in the country. It also uses the most pesticides in the country.

SPECIAL INTEREST

Cancer is often the last stage of a degenerative process in the body. Most carcinogens have an effect on the regulatory system in the body, such as the central nervous system, through neurotransmittors, hormones, and the immune system. We are now seeing the first host of other problems, such as learning disabilities, hyperactivity in children, increased infections across all ages, asthma, a whole slew of neurological diseases, cardiovascular and hormonal disturbances, as well as bone/collagen problems. Generally, environmental factors, diet and nutritional deficiencies, have been slow in being considered as having anything to do with these health problems. Instead of instituting true preventative measures, billions of dollars are spent for early diagnosis, for pharmaceutical and/or invasive technologies and therapies. Cancer is still not "cured," while our "health care" budget is not the bottomless pit it seems to be.

The budget for cancer treatment in the USA was $170 million in 1971, $3 billion in 2000, and it continues to rise. President Clinton, while in office, increased the budget to $5 billion by 2003. Survival rates are no different than in the 1950s.

We can't wait for preventive measures to be instituted by government, industry, corporations or other organizations. Individuals can start at home. Wider change will be encouraged through the very real power that consumers have. **Buy healthy, buy green, buy non-toxic!** Do this for yourself, your families, your loved ones, and for all children. Arm yourself with knowledge, hope and perseverance. If you're an activist type, get active! The good news is: prevention works, and works best before conception.

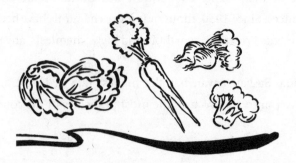

PREVENTION AT HOME

Kitchen

PRODUCT SOURCES	PROBLEMS/CHEMICALS	CORRECTIVE/PREVEN-TATIVE MEASURES
Fruits, vegetables	95% dioxins and furans; sixty carcinogenic pesticides used in production; pesticides, herbicides, organochlorines, organophosphates	Switch to organic produce as much as possible. "Perfect" looking produce isn't healthier. Eat foods high in antioxidants. Wash all produce thoroughly, whether organic or not. However, washing or peeling will not remove pesticides completely.
Dairy products	Hormone disrupting chemicals (xenoestrogens): PCB, DDT, etc.	Reduce consumption of milk, cream and cheese. Buy organic.
Meats	Hormones, antibiotics	Eliminate fatty meats. Avoid USA beef (contains bovine growth hormone). Buy organic.
Fish from industrial waterways or fish farms	Xenoestrogens, cadmium. mercury, antibiotics	Freshwater fish from clean areas, small fish (lower on the food chain).
Diets high in fats, high in carbohydrates	Fat-soluble chemicals and solvents	Organic lean meats, organic dairy products, fibre (vegetable).
Chlorinated water	Trihalomethanes (chloroform)	Charcoal or reverse osmosis filtrations; glass-bottled spring water from a safe source
Food colours, preservatives	Dyes, particularly Red dye #3	Organic food, homemade food; read labels
Plastic containers, styrene cups, can liners, Teflon cookware	Xenoestrogens: PVC, alkylphenols, nonyphenols, bisphenol A, phthalates	Glass containers, stainless steel, ceramic, cast iron, glassware, paper cups, fresh foods. Never heat any product in plastic in a microwave or oven.
Oven cleaners	Solvents	Baking soda, self-cleaning ovens (non-catalytic), non-toxic products

SPECIAL INTEREST

PRODUCT SOURCES	PROBLEMS/CHEMICALS	CORRECTIVE/PREVEN-TATIVE MEASURES
Gas stoves	Organic volatile compounds	Electric stove with vented hood to the outside
Laminated countertops	Formaldehyde, VOCs outgassing from unfinished underside	Laminate underneath as well or permanently apply foil to seal. Granite, wood, marble, Corian, stainless steel are better choices
Microwaves	Electromagnetic field (EMF)	If you really want to use these, keep 3 feet away from microwave when cooking; keep stored foods and vitamins out of vicinity

Bedrooms

PRODUCT SOURCES	PROBLEMS/CHEMICALS	CORRECTIVE/PREVEN-TATIVE MEASURES
Electric blankets, pads, water beds	Electromagnetic field (EMF)	Box mattress set or futon from natural materials
Foam mattresses, pillows	Styrene	Cotton, wool, feather, down
Geopathic stress	EMF radiation due to rocks under tension or running streams, under building	Locate by dowsing, place beds in safe spot
Synthetic carpeting with or without adhesives	Volatile Organic Compounds (VOCs), pesticides	Hardwood, natural-fibre area rugs
Wallpaper	Mold retarding pesticides, vinyl covering	Low VOC paint over plaster or drywall
Mothballs	VOCs	Cedarwood (chips, eggs, chests) unless sensitive to cedar
Dry cleaning	Perchloroethylene, tetrachloroethylene	Water cleaning–"green" dry cleaners offer this
Children's toys	Vinyls, plastics (use your nose–if the toy smells, throw it out)	Wooden toys
Scented markers	toluene	Water-based, fragrance-free markers

Bathrooms

PRODUCT SOURCES	PROBLEMS/CHEMICALS	CORRECTIVE/PREVEN-TATIVE MEASURES
Lotions, creams	Di- and tri-ethanolamines with nitrites as preservative produce nitrozamines	Preservative-free natural products
Hair colouring	Dark brown/black dyes: phenylenediamines	Hennas, vegetable dyes
Head lice shampoos (p. 220)	Lindane (organochlorine)	Vinegar, olive oil, tea tree oil, lavender and rosemary essential oils
Nailpolish	Solvents	Use in well-ventilated areas, read labels—avoid toluene particularly
Spermicides, vaginal gels	Nonyphenols	If not sensitive, use latex or sheepskin condoms; natural method: Billings Ovulation Method, Creighton Model Fertility Care System www.naprotechnology.com

Garage/Basements/Laundry

PRODUCT SOURCES	PROBLEMS/CHEMICALS	CORRECTIVE/PREVEN-TATIVE MEASURES
Garage under living space (houses, apartments)	Petroleum products, VOCs	If unavoidable, ensure good seals, ventilation, air filtration at home. Attached or separate garage preferable.
Storage of paints, solvents, pesticides, herbicides, waxes, gasoline	VOCs, benzene, toluene, hormone disruptors	Avoid use of pesticides and herbicides. Store anything toxic out of the house. Even garages should have some ventilation.
Gas, oil heating	VOCs	Electric, high efficiency gas, solar heating, ground heat pumps

SPECIAL INTEREST

PRODUCT SOURCES	PROBLEMS/CHEMICALS	CORRECTIVE/PREVEN-TATIVE MEASURES
Cleaning agents, polishes, varnishes, domestic aerosols, fabric softeners, liquid laundry detergents	Solvents	Baking soda, borax, vinegar, "green" products
Cat litter filler, flea collars	Crystalline silica, dichlorovos	Read labels, use "green" products

Recreation

PRODUCT SOURCES	PROBLEMS/CHEMICALS	CORRECTIVE/PREVEN-TATIVE MEASURES
Lawns, gardens, golf courses, parks	Herbicides, 2, 4-D, Roundup: linked to cancers and neurological disorders	Organic lawn care
Old utility poles/railway ties	Pentachlorophenols, dioxin, furans	Do not use in gardens
Sports fields under high tension power lines	EMF	Don't play or walk under high tension wires
Gas fireplaces, space heater, wood smoke	VOCs	Avoid gas or kerosene space heaters; seal fireplaces tight
Hobby paints, glues, epoxy, stripping	Solvents	Safe water-soluble furniture glues, nontoxic strippers and paints
Tobacco smoking, bingo parlors, bars, second-hand smoke	2000 chemicals, including benzopyrene, known to cause lung cancer	Avoid smoking and exposure to second-hand smoke, ban smoking at home, even by guests and family members
Alcohol	Ethyl alcohol or ethanol	Education, involvement in sports and/or other activities
Indoor ice rinks–gas powered Zambonis	VOCs (benzene, toluene), carbon monoxide	Avoid being at rink during or soon after use

Medical Procedures/Medications

PRODUCT SOURCES	PROBLEMS/CHEMICALS	CORRECTIVE/PREVEN-TATIVE MEASURES
X-rays, mammograms (especially before menopause)	X-ray radiation	Use thermography instead. If mammography used take antioxidants before and after, particularly CoQ10
I.V. bags, I.V delivery system	PVC (polyvinyl chloride)	PVC-free I.V. bags, glass containers
Tagamet (cimetidine–ulcer therapy); Pravachol (pravastatin–cholesterol lowering drug)	Estrogenic effect	Substitute
Prozac, Elabil (antidepressants)	Promotes breast cancer in rodents	Substitute
Haloperidol (antipsychotic)	Increases secretion of prolactin and linked to increased breast cancer in rodents	Substitute
Valium (diazepam– tranquilizer, antianxiety)	Increases prolactin, a hormone known to stimulate the growth and development of invasive breast cancer	Substitute
Xanax (alprazolam– tranquilizer, antianxiety)	May increase invasiveness of undiagnosed cancer	Substitute
All anti-cancer drugs	Used for cancer therapy; are themselves carcinogenic	Have anti-oxidant I.V. after chemotherapy
Flagyl (metronidazole– antibacterial, antiprotozoal)	Linked to breast cancer	Substitute
Tenormin (atenolol– betablocker)	Linked to breast & pituitary cancer in rodents	Substitute
Aldactone (spironolactone– antihypertensive)	Linked to increased breast cancer in rodents	Substitute
Apresoline (hydralazine– antihypertensive)	Linked to increased risk of breast cancer	Substitute

SPECIAL INTEREST

PRODUCT SOURCES	PROBLEMS/CHEMICALS	CORRECTIVE/PREVEN-TATIVE MEASURES
Serpasil (reserpine–antihypertensive)	Increases prolactin	Substitute
Oral contraceptive tablets (1st and 2nd generation tablets–estrogen)	Linked to breast cancer	If not sensitive, use latex or sheepskin condoms, natural method: Billings Ovulation Method, Creighton Model Fertility Care System www.naprotechnology.com
Menopausal hormone replacement (estrogens)	Linked to 30 to 70% increase in breast cancer	Substitute with natural estrogen, herbs. Progesterone alone may solve problem. If family history of breast, uterine or ovarian cancer, stay off estrogen.

ELECTROMAGNETIC RADIATION (EMR)

It is impossible not to mention, briefly, a very complicated but real phenomenon of the effect of EMR on humans, and particularly on chemically sensitive people. Human-created EMR is many times greater than naturally occurring electromagnetic fields. Domestic electricity devices operate at 60 hertz (Hz) in the US and Canada, and at 50 Hz in Europe, Japan and Russia. It is believed that exposure to 60 Hz creates more health problems than exposure to 50 Hz

EMR is an energy that travels and spreads in the form of waves out of the many gadgets that modern technology has cre-

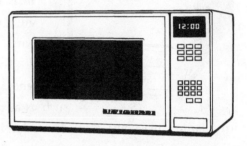

ated. Waves of EMR can be divided into visible waves such as light from lamps, sun; audible waves such various radio waves and waves which are neither visible nor audible, such as microwaves, infrared, ultraviolet light, x-rays and gamma rays.

In general, radio waves are characterized by low frequency and long waves. X-rays and gamma rays have high frequency and short waves. The visible spectrum of light is in between, which is most natural and is safe for most

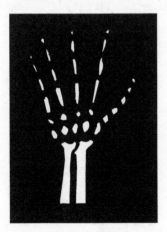

species, including humans. The waves on either side of the visual spectrum of light are known to produce health problems. e.g., effects of x-ray waves or microwaves. There are also extreme low frequency waves (ELF), which cause many clinical problems.

There are some individuals who develop sensitivity to EMR. They are usually very ill, chemically intoxicated, nutritionally deprived, and generally very maladapted individuals, who are bothered by everything in their diet, work and home environment. They are not mentally ill as assumed by most doctors and even family. They are most difficult to treat. They can develop

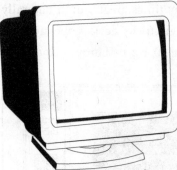

bizarre symptoms in the presence of microwaves, radios, cellphones, computers, television sets, radar equipment and/or antennas, electric blankets, water beds and many other electrically operating gadgets, as well as high-tension wires.

There are not only a number of documented symptoms from these patients, such as anxiety depression, insomnia, heart irregularities, blackouts, severely swollen limbs, dizziness, headaches, but also serious diseases such as heart disorders and cancer, particularly different forms of leukemias. According to Andrew Michrowski, PhD (see Resources), who carries out electromagnetic surveys of buildings and farms, 70% of a building's electromagnetic pollution problem is related to wiring errors, faulty grounding and net current between live wires and water pipes.

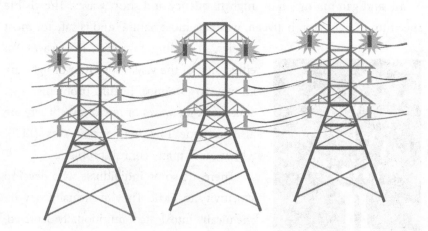

NUCLEAR RADIATION

ANOTHER PIECE OF THE TOTAL LOAD PUZZLE – JUST HOW SAFE IS IT?

Most of the time, the health effects of nuclear radiation are measured and discussed in terms of cancer only. Other effects, such as cellular damage, chronic or mental illness, are often completely overlooked.

Since the first discovery of radium (a radioactive metal) by Marie Sklodowska Curie in 1911, there has been a continuous and ever bigger development of the nuclear industry through the creation of isotopes. X-ray technology in nuclear medicine for diagnosis and treatment has led to hundreds of thousands of individuals being exposed in medical and veterinary practice.

The first use of nuclear weapons occurred in 1945 on Hiroshima and Nagasaki, with atmospheric nuclear bomb testing beginning in 1946 by the USA, followed by the Soviet Union in 1949, England in 1950, and continued by France, China, India and Pakistan, until 1998. **This has created immense global pollution and internal radioactive contamination.** Over two thousand nuclear explosions or tests around the world have taken place since that fateful day of August 6, 1945.

These events have led to a military policy dependent on nuclear weaponry. This basic fact has led to a mushrooming of uranium mining, milling and processing facilities, production of nuclear reactors and weapons, reprocessing facilities and hundreds of transportation activities, as well as waste storage sites associated with each of these industries.

Each of these industries carries the hazards of real and potential major disasters, such as the well-known Three Mile Island in 1979 and Chernobyl in 1986. There continues to be, into the foreseeable future, widespread use of Depleted Uranium (DU) by the US military in bullets, artillery shells and missile warheads.

DU is a waste product from the process that produces uranium used in atomic weapons and nuclear power plants. Apparently it is so plentiful, it is given away to arms manufacturers. It is toxic and radioactive with a half-life of 4.5 <u>billion</u> years (no, not a misprint). It is extremely dense and pyrophoric, which means it is easily combustible, as when striking steel. When DU burns (as it does on impact), it discharges radioactive uranium oxide in aerosol form. Because of the extremely high temperature on impact, these particles become like glass. They can be carried for miles with the wind. It is in this form, able to be inhaled and almost insoluble in body fluid, causing it to be retained by the body for a long time and irradiating the surrounding cells, that it is becoming dangerous.

DU was massively used (at least 40 tonnes) during the Gulf War in Iraq, Kuwait and Saudi Arabia, contaminating hundreds of square miles of southern Iraq and northern Kuwait. The same DU was used in Kosovo and most likely in Afghanistan. There have been many reports of medical problems among troops who served in these wars, including respiratory, liver and kidney dysfunction, memory loss, headaches, fever, low blood pressure and even birth defects among their newborn children. Generally the health problems have been attributed to "post-traumatic stress disorder." Exposure is compared with that of uranium dust, which is not the same as a ceramic aerosol form.

The assessment of the health effects of these pollutants is always dismissive or secretive and hidden from the public, so as to be able to portray nuclear energy as "clean and safe."

The field of radiation and its health effects are presently studied and controlled by mathematicians, physicists, engineers and radiology technicians instead of by physicians, epidemiologists and biologists. Often, in response to demand for health studies, governments will organize studies headed by psychiatrists who describe symptoms from radioactive exposure as "radiophobia" or as a purely psychological phenomenon.

There is a continuous debate about the recommendations of an "allowable dose" for the protection of workers' health and the health of the general public among America, Britain and other nations. After a formal petition submitted to the International Commission of Radiological Protection, pressure from more than seven hundred scientists and physicians, among other pressures, recommended worker exposure was reduced and established at 2 rad (20 mSv) per year, and exposure for the public was also considerably reduced to 0.1 rad (1 mSv) per year. This recommendation refers to each source of nuclear radiation. In the United States, after legal action to reduce exposures, nuclear radiation from a local facility can cause exposures of no more than 0.02 mSv, because the individual will receive exposure from other sources more distant through air, water and food movement. *[1 rad is roughly comparable to two major trunk x-ray examinations, and 0.1 rad would about double the radiation which a person receives from terrestrial and cosmic sources over a year.]*

Some geneticists continue to oppose extension of nuclear technology to the civilian population. A. B. Bridges has suggested that the radiation dose for genetic mutations cannot be predicted. Most of the radiation effects for acute and close exposure are known as radiation sickness and include nausea, vomiting, diarrhea, hair loss and a decrease of blood cells. The effect of alteration of cells and their DNA leads to cancer.

We are only beginning to know more about the low level effect of radiation:

- Rudi Nussbaum reports on miscarriages, Trisomy 21 (Down's) syndrome, stillbirths, neuroblastoma, neonatal hypothyroidism and other mutations due to low dose radioactivity.
- The same author relates low doses of ionizing radiation to cancer, mutational effects among radiotherapy technicians, increased infant mortality rate, increased low birth weights and premature births after exposure.
- Permitted effluence from even normally operating nuclear facilities may not be safe. A Columbia University radiation study concludes that there is no safe level of radiation. Even a single particle of radiation can induce mutations and chromosome aberrations in cells that receive direct radiation to their DNA.
- Accidental exposures to x-ray radiation are dangerous to x-ray technicians and patients, especially during pregnancy.

SPECIAL INTEREST

- There are reports of childhood cancers in the United Kingdom related to background radiation.
- Radiation causes general cell depression of the developing brain, leading to small heads (microencephaly) and mental retardation.
- The Chernobyl accident and follow-up effects are well researched and described.
- Radioactive strontium 90 can replace calcium, leading to bone deformities and causing damage to blood stem cells, causing a variety of hematological problems (anemias, cancers, etc.)
- Radioactive iodine causes both hypo- and hyper- thyroidism and especially Hashimoto's thyroiditis (inflammation of the thyroid). Radioactive Cesium (137) can displace sodium from the cell, particularly in the muscles of heart and skeletal muscles, causing an epidemic of cardiac insufficiency, muscle spasms and severe pain.
- A decrease in monocyte stem cells causes iron deficiency anemia, since monocytes recycle about 37% of the heme from dead red blood cells.
- In Belarus (a former Russian republic), the fallout from the Chernobyl disaster was heaviest, and the effect of radioactive cesium was researched carefully by Dr. Y. Bandazevsky (a pathologist) and his wife (a cardiac pediatrician). They coined the term "Cesium Cardiomyopathy," in which cardiac damage becomes irreversible. Sudden death can occur anytime, including in children. For his efforts in doing this research, Dr. Bandazevsky was arrested by a presidential decree aimed at fighting "terrorism." Amnesty International has listed him as a prisoner of conscience. Many Russian, Ukrainian and Belarussian scientists have been silenced in international circles by their respective governments. (See Bibliography)

HOSPITAL ADMISSIONS FOR PATIENTS WITH ENVIRONMENTAL HYPERSENSITIVITY DISORDER

There are times when a hospital admission is necessary for any number of reasons. However, until an environmental control unit becomes available in every hospital, the following precautions are recommended for the highly sensitive. In varying degrees, they can help any hospitalized patient avoid further problems and improve the chances of good recovery. Hospitalization is a humbling experience at best. The environmentally hypersensitive, however, besides facing whatever ailment brings them to a hospital, additionally often face an attitude of disbelief on the part of hospital staff regarding their sensitivities that, according to reports of some patients, borders on psychological abuse. To avoid this situation, which is hardly conducive to a recovery, patients must ask their physician to give written instructions to the hospital medical staff, outlining the patient's needs in the following areas:

- A description of the nature and severity of the sensitivity
- A list of substances and/or medications to which the patient reacts adversely
- A suggestion that the patient may have additional information to offer
- A recommendation to treat adverse reactions seriously; they are not psychological in nature and may result in serious complications if dismissed, the responsibility for the consequences of which must then be borne by the staff.

The patient's physician should offer to be available for additional discussion.

Additionally, depending, of course, on the degree and severity of the sensitivity, the following requests could be made:

- A private room, preferably not carpeted (yes, it's hard to believe, but some hospitals actually carpet patient rooms—not only off-gassing problems but thoroughly unhygenic as well!)

- A private bathroom, preferably
- Patients to be allowed to remove any offending substances from the room if detected by their (typically) acute sense of smell.
- Ensure good ventilation and environmental control
- The patient to use his/her own toiletries, bedding, water, portable air filter, if necessary
- The room to be mopped first, before others (to avoid bringing contaminants in) and only with water or safe cleaning products

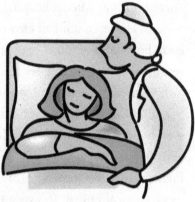

- No one who has recently smoked or is wearing clothing impregnated with the smell of tobacco to be allowed near the patient
- No perfumes or scents of any kind to be used by anyone in contact with the patient, including physicians, nurses, cleaners, or visitors
- No visitors or staff who have had contact with animals
- Posting adverse reactions on a bedside chart for easy referral by staff
- No waxing, painting or smoking in the vicinity of the patient's room

If the admission is not on an emergency basis, it would be a good idea for the hypersensitive patient with a friend or member of the family to:

- Visit the hospital ahead of time and speak with the nursing supervisor and maintenance staff about the matter of sensitivity. This is also a good time to deliver a copy of the attending physician's letter.
- Visit with the dietitian to arrange any special menus or the possibility of storing and preparing the patient's own tolerated foods.
- Consult with the hospital pharmacist to discuss medication with few fillers and colours.

The following are more recommendations for treating, clearing and avoiding adverse reactions. (In the case of anaphylaxis, however, the standard hospital protocol of therapy must be used first to stabilize the patient):

- Oxygen can be administered at 4–6 L/minute for 20 minutes. Ask for a ceramic mask, not the soft plastic ones usually used. (I remember one patient in hospital who was adversely reacting even when getting oxygen. I switched her to a ceramic mask, and the patient settled down. The attending resident asked me what the difference in the masks was. I told him to use his nose to compare odours. Two sniffs answered his question.)
- Alka-Seltzer Gold (without aspirin) salts can be tried orally
- Natrium bicarbonate as an I.V. works well for many individuals
- 7–14 gms of vitamin C as an I.V. is often very helpful
- The patient will need permission to use his/her own injections
- For any I.V. drips, normal saline or Ringer's lactate causes fewer problems than a dextrose-in-water solution
- Both local and general anesthetics can be problematic, but there is no way to avoid them, one can only minimize reactions. Nevertheless, if possible, avoid hydrocarbon gases.

Dr. William Rea, a cardiovascular surgeon, as well as an expert in Environmental Medicine in Dallas Texas, makes the following suggestions in his book, *Chemical Sensitivity*, Volume 4, for operation premedication:

- Benadryl and an atropine sulphite injection are usually tolerated. It is helpful to administrate 100% oxygen for five minutes prior to inducing anesthesia with thiopental sodium (penthatol). Succinylcholine chloride (Anectine) and fentanyl citrate (Sublimaze) are usually acceptable and sufficient to obliterate memory and provide anesthesia.
- With proper awareness and arrangements, patients with even severe environmental sensitivities can have a safe and tolerable stay in hospital. (See Bibliography)

Appendix: Protocols

This appendix includes information *regarding actual treatment protocols used by Dr. Krop and other physicians only after careful assessment and diagnosis of individual patients. These protocols are periodically adjusted. The information in this appendix is not intended as therapeutic advice. Do not administer these treatments to yourself or others. Discuss these treatments with your physician.*

DENTAL AMALGAM REPLACEMENT FOR ADULTS: NUTRIENT SUPPLEMENT PROTOCOL

Never replace amalgams shortly before or during pregnancy or lactation. Dentists trained in amalgam replacement usually provide very good mechanical protection (rubber dam, mask, oxygen, ionizer removing mercury vapour). Amalgam replacement requires intensive nutritional supplementation in order to protect individuals from re-intoxication with mercury during the dental procedure. **Compatability for dental materials can be assessed prior to amalgam replacement.** Additional biological/nutritional protection is recommended.

Stage I-4 weeks before amalgam replacement:

1. Vitamin C: 1 gram 3 times per day (discontinue 24 hours before procedure if you plan on using anesthetic)
2. B complex, high potency: 1 capsule, twice per day
3. Multiminerals, broad spectrum: 1–2 capsules, 3 times per day
4. Selenium, liquid: 1 tsp, twice per day or one 200 mcg capsule twice per day
5. Methionine and taurine (e.g., Redoxal): 500 mg, 3 times per day
6. N-acetylcysteine 500 mg 2 × / day or glutathione (e.g., Oxygard) 1 capsule 2 × / day
7. Lipoic acid 100 mg 2 times per day
8. High-protein diet

Stage II—20 minutes before removal, take 750 mg activated charcoal tablets.

Stage III—On the day of the procedure and for 3 days after, continue Stage I with the following changes/additions:

1. Increase vitamin C to 2 grams, 3 times per day (some dentisits provide I.V. vitamin C during the procedure)
2. Garlic 3–4 capsules, 3 times per day
3. Lentils (soup or salad), 3 times per day
4. Continue steps 2, 3, 4, 5,6 and 7 from Stage I
5. On the fourth day, discontinue or decrease garlic and lentils.
6. On the 8th day after the procedure, return to Stage I only and continue for 2–3 weeks. If you have another dental replacement session **within** this time period, restart Stage 1 and continue to Stage 3.

Repeat this protocol **each time** you are having amalgams replaced.

Patients not tolerating nutrients orally may be able to tolerate them by intravenous method after testing the ingredients for sensitivity. Vitamin C with DMPS can be given intravenously immediately after the procedure.

Chemically sensitive and fragile patients should not replace more than two amalgams at one time and may need a longer interval between sessions (more than one month).

Ideally, after the final amalgam replacement, a chelation challenge test for mercury and other heavy metals is recommended. If the test is positive, chelation therapy for heavy metals is indicated.

CHALLENGE TEST FOR HEAVY METALS IN CHILDREN

This test is recommended for children with developmental delay, ADHD and Autistic Spectrum Disorder. Before using any of the following substances, electrodermal screening for tolerance to all ingredients is suggested.

	CHILD 2– 5 YEARS	CHILD 6 YEARS & OVER
Methionine, taurine (e.g., Redoxal)	½ capsule 2 x per day (6 wks)	1 capsule 2 x per day (10wks)
Glutathione (e.g., Oxygard)	½ capsule 2 x per day (6 wks)	1 capsule 2 x per day (10 wks)
B complex	1 capsule once per day (6 wks)	1 capsule 2 x per day (10 wks)
Vitamin C	250 mg. capsule 2 x per day (6 wks)	500 mg. capsule 2 x per day (10 wks)
Selenium liquid 200 mcg/ 5cc (none on DMSA/LA and DMPS days)	½ tspn 1 x per day (6 wks)	½–1 tspn 1 x per day (10 wks)
Homeopathic EDTA (e.g., Metoxsol)	5–10 drops 3 x per day/15cc of water (6 wks)	10 drops 3 x per day/15 cc of water (10 wks)
Multiminerals (none on DMSA/LA and DMPS days)	1 capsule per day (6 wks) (none on DMSA/LA and DMPS days)	1 capsule 2 x per day (10 wks) (none on DMSA/LA and DMPS days)
DMSA 10 mg/kg, 3 x per day Alpha lipoic acid (LA) 2 mg/kg, 3 x per day	Take above vitamins for 11 days. On day 12, 13, 14 add DMSA and LA . Repeat 3 times (6 weeks)	Take above vitamins for 11 days. On day 12, 13, 14 add DMSA and LA. Repeat 5 times (10 weeks)
DMPS injection (3mg/kilo) in physician office followed by 24 or 6 hour urine collection	Immediately after 3rd repeat of DMSA/LA capsules, go to physician for DMPS injection	Immediately after 5th repeat of DMSA/LA capsules, go to physician for DMPS injection

For the ensuing urinalysis, note the time of the DMPS injection and begin to collect urine in the container provided by your physician for the next 24 (or 6) hours as directed. Do not let the child urinate directly into container (there is acid in the container that may splash back). After completing the collection, record the total amount of urine collected (measures are noted on side of container). Shake the container for 15 seconds and fill the provided urine sample cup. On the cup label, write patient name, date and total amount of urine collected, as well as number of hours. Close tightly and bring or send by courier to your physician, who will send it on to the appropriate laboratory for analysis.

CHELATION THERAPY FOR HEAVY METALS IN CHILDREN

(1 month = 28 days)

Before using any of the following substances, electrodermal screening for tolerance to all ingredients is suggested.

	CHILD 2-5 YEARS	CHILD 6 YEARS & OVER
Methionine, taurine (e.g., Redoxal)	½ capsule 2 x per day (1 mo.)	1 capsule 2 x per day (1 mo.)
Glutathione (e.g., Oxygard)	⅓ capsule 2 x per day (1 mo.)	1 capsule 2 x per day (1 mo.)
B complex	1 capsule once per day (1 mo.)	1 capsule 2 x per day (1 mo.)
Vitamin C	250 mg. capsule 2 x per day (1 mo.)	500 mg. capsule 2 x per day (1 mo.)
Selenium liquid 200 mcg/ 5cc (none on DMSA, LA and DMPS days)	½ tspn 1 x per day (1 mo.)	½–1 tspn 1 x per day (1 mo.)
Homeopathic EDTA (e.g., Metoxsol)	5-10 drops 3 x per day/ 15cc of water (1 mo.)	10 drops 3 x per day/15 cc of water (1 mo.)
Multiminerals (none on DMSA, LA and DMPS days)	1 capsule once per day (1 mo.) (BUT none on DMSA and DMPS days)	1 capsule 2 x per day (1 mo.) (BUT none on DMSA and DMPS days)
Alpha lipoic acid(LA) 2 mg/kg, 3 x per day	Start on 11th day for 3 days	Start on 11th day for 3 days
DMSA 10 mg/kg, 3 x per day	Start on 11th day for 3 days	Start on 11th day for 3 days
	Continue taking vitamins and minerals for another 11 days	Continue taking vitamins and minerals for another 11 days
	On 25th day, restart alpha lipoic acid and DMSA for 3 days	On 25th day, restart alpha lipoic acid and DMSA for 3 days
DMPS Injection in the office	On the 28th day (immediately after DMSA), come to office	On the 28th day (immediately after DMSA), come to office

This one-month treatment should be repeated eight times. In the eighth month, a 6 or 24-hour urine collection will be repeated. Blood for hematology, liver and kidney functions should be checked regularly.

ADULT CHELATION CHALLENGE TEST FOR HEAVY METALS
(Patient should be amalgam-free)

1. Electrodermal screening for tolerance to all ingredients is recommended

2. Start with the following:
   Vitamin C 1000 mg 2–3 × / day for 14 days
   B complex vitamins (25–50 mg) 2 capsules / day for 14 days
   Selenium liquid 1 tspn. 2 × / day
   Multiminerals (broad spectrum) 2 × / day for 10 days
   Methionine and taurine (e.g., Redoxal) 500 mg each 2 × / day for 14 days
   N-acetylcysteine 500 mg 2 × / day or glutathione (e.g., Oxygard)
   500 mg 2 × / day for 14 days
   Alpha lipoic acid 100 mg 3 × / day for 14 days
   Homéopathic EDTA (e.g., Metoxsol) 10 drops 3 × / day for 14 days

3. On the eleventh day, stop the multiminerals and selenium only and additionally start to take:
   DMSA 500 mg twice per day for 4 days

4. On the 15th day get a DMPS I.V. and a 24-hour urine collection test, which will measure any heavy metal levels.

Note the time the DMPS I.V. is finished and begin to collect urine in the container provided to you for the next 24 hours. Do not urinate directly into the container (acid is in the container that may splash back). After completing the collection, record the total amount of urine collected (measures are noted on the side of the container). Shake the container for

APPENDIX

15 seconds and fill the urine sample cup (also provided). You may discard the rest of the urine. On the urine sample cup label, write patient name, date and total amount of urine collected. Close the sample cup tightly and bring or send by courier to your physician, who will send it on to the appropriate laboratory for analysis.

TREATMENT FOR MERCURY/HEAVY METALS TOXICITY IN ADULTS

Treatment is cycled over an 8 month period. This protocol should be administered and supervised only by a physician. Electrodermal screening for tolerance to supplements is recommended.

Day 1–7

Vitamin C 1 gram 3 × / day

B complex hi-potency (25–50 mg) 1 capsule 2 × / day

Selenium liquid 1 tspn. / day

Multiminerals (broad spectrum) 2 capsules 2 × / day

Methionine and taurine (e.g., Redoxal) 500 mg each 2 × / day

N-acetylcysteine 500 mg 2 × / day or glutathione (e.g., Oxygard) 1 cap.
    2 × / day

Homeopathic EDTA (e.g., Metoxsol): 10 drops in two tblspns. of water
    3 × / day

Day 8–14

Continue supplements as for Day 1–7 and, in addition:

Start lipoic acid 200 mg 2 × / day and DMSA 500 mg 2 × / day
    on day 11 for 4 days only*

* *Do not take multiminerals or selenium on these 4 days*

Day 15—21
Continue supplements as for days 1—7

Day 22—28
Continue supplements as for days 1—7 and, in addition:
Start lipoic acid 200 mg 2 × / day and DMSA 500 mg 2 × / day **on day 24
    for 4 days only***

Day 28*: DMPS I.V. 250 mg (5 cc) with Vitamin C 5 gm (10 cc)
* Do not take multiminerals or selenium on these five days

Repeat this 4-week cycle **8 times**. Blood for hematology, liver and kidney functions should be checked regularly.

At the end of the treatment cycle, a 24-hour urine collection test should be ordered to check the heavy metal level. Occasionally, instead of less, higher levels are found. This can occur if an individual has been heavily intoxicated, or individual metabolism has been unable to excrete newly mobilized heavy metals out of tissues adequately, and treatment should be continued.

COLLAGEN DISEASE PROTOCOL (RHEUMATOID ARTHRITIS, SCLERODERMA, ETC.)

Intravenous Clindamycin 300 mg.

Day 1 and 2:   300 mg (1 ampoule) in 50 cc of normal saline or sterile water over one hour

Day 3 and 4:   600 mg (2 ampoules) in 150 cc of normal saline or sterile water over one hour

Day 5:   900 mg (3 ampoules) in 200 cc of normal saline or sterile water over one hour

Thereafter: 900 mg in 200 cc of normal saline or sterile water over one hour, **once per week for 8 consecutive weeks.**

After the first week, start 100 mg. Doxycyline orally, 1 or two tablets, depending on tolerance, 3 times per week (Monday, Wednesday, Friday) **or**
100 mg Minocin orally, 1 or two tablets depending on tolerance, 3 times per week (M,W,F)

This oral treatment can be continued for at least one half year or longer. Protect the gastrointestinal tract with probiotics and antifungal medications.

INTRAVENOUS PROTOCOLS

CONDITIONS: INGREDIENTS:	CV ATHEROSCLEROSIS	CV ATHEROSCLEROSIS ↑CREATININE	ARRYTHMIAS OR CFS	CFS, NEGATIVE FOR PROLACTIN	NUTRITIONAL	MERCURY INTOXICATION[4]	AMALGAM REPLACEMENT	PORPHYRIA	ACUTE VIRAL INFECTIONS[5] E.G. HERPES
Sterile H2O	500 cc					250 cc		250 or 500 cc	500 cc
Nl Saline 0.9%			250 cc		250 cc				
½ N Saline 0.45%				125 cc					
Ringer's Lactate							500 cc		
Water/Dextrose 5%		250 cc							
Dextrose 50%, 500 mg/cc								50-100 cc	
Vit C-500 mg/cc	20 cc		10 cc	10 cc	20 cc	20 cc	40-60 cc	20-30 cc	40-60 cc
Plaquex[1] 500 mg/10cc		10 cc							
EDTA 150 mg/cc[2]	-20 cc								
DMPS 50 mg/cc						5 cc push (at the end of the I.V.)			
Glutathione[3] 600mg						600 mg			1000 mg
Amino Acids: 12 + 8				125 cc					
Lysine[3] 100 0 mg									
Co-Enzyme Q10			300 mg						
Heparin 1000 μ/cc	2 cc		2 cc						
Na Bicarb 84 mg/cc	10 cc		10 cc		10 cc	10 cc		1-1.5 cc	10 cc
Calcium 100 mg/cc	5 cc				5 cc			10 cc	
Mag 500 mg/cc	5 cc		10 cc	5 cc	5 cc	5 cc			
KCl 2 meq/cc	5 cc		5 cc	5 cc		5 cc	5 cc	10 cc	
B-Complex 25 or 100 mg/cc	2 cc or 1 cc		2 cc or 1 cc	2 cc or 1 cc	2 cc or 1 cc			1 cc of 100 mg/cc	
B12 1000 μg/cc	1 cc		1 cc		1 cc			1 cc	
Folic Acid 5 mg/cc	1 cc		1 cc		1 cc				
D-Pan 250 mg/cc					1 cc			1 cc	
B6 100 mg/cc					1 cc			1 cc	
Selenium 40 μg/cc							3 cc		
Minerals-MTE 5					1 cc				

[1] Plaquex (phosphatidylcholine, deoxycholic acid, Vitamin E, adenosine-5 triphosphate, nicotinic acid)

[2] Calculated on the basis of Cockcroft-Gault equation

[3] In powder form reconstituted and the solution must be sterilized through a bacterial micro-filter (0.22 microns)

[4] given 1 x per month preceded by oral detoxification

[5] This procedure is most effective when combined with SDEPT neutralization using fluogen vaccine

NOTE: All ingredients should be screened for tolerance. The easiest method is electrodermal. B-Complex particularly can be problematic for some patients causing nausea and even vomiting. In that case, omit or choose a substitute.

Resources

GENERAL

Canada Mortgage and Housing
  Corporation (CMHC)
700 Montreal Road
Ottawa, Ontario K1A 0P7
The Clean Air Guide—excellent
information for homeowner to
better air quality
Order from: 1-800-668-2642
(outside Canada, call 613-748-2003)
www.cmhc-schl.gc.ca
• CMHC offers a wealth of information for
  healthy building and renovating.

The Canadian Lung Association
1750 Courtwood Crescent,
Suite 300, Ottawa, ON, K2C 2B5,
(613)-569-6411
Fax: 613-569-8860
1-888-566-LUNG for questions on
lung health
• Dedicated to improving respiratory
  health: "When you can't breathe
  nothing else matters." Many positive

programs including the Quit Smoking
Guide and C.A.N. DO program linking
health to air quality. Practical resources:
clean air home audit, in depth fact sheets.
Contact your Provincial Lung Association
to order C.A.N. DO materials.
www.lung.ca
www.lung.ca/cando

Canadian Environmental Law
  Association,
130 Spadina Avenue, Suite 301,
Toronto, ON M5V 2L4
416-960-2284
Fax: 416-960-9392
www.cela.ca
• A non-profit, public interest organization
  using existing laws to protect the
  environment and advocate environmental
  law reforms. Also a free legal advisory
  clinic for the public. Publications
  available online.

International Institute of Concern
   for Public Health
P.O. Box 80523 Rpo White Shields
2300 Lawrence Ave. East
Toronto ON Canada M1P 4Z5
416-755-3685
www.iicph.org
• Nonprofit organization helps
  communities assess environmental
  health status, alerts and informs public
  of health hazards of pesticides, nuclear
  industries and other commercial, military and industrial products.

Friends of the Earth
260 St. Patrick Street, Suite 300
Ottawa, Ontario, K1N 5K5,
(613) 241-0085
1-888-385-4444
Fax: (613) 241-7998
E-Mail **foe@forcanada.org**
www.foecanada.org
• National voice for the environment
  through research, education and advocacy.

Friends of the Earth International
www.foei.org

Pollution Probe
625 Church St., Suite 402
Toronto, ON M4Y 2G1
416-926-1907
Fax: 416-926-1601
www.pollutionprobe.org
• For over 30 years this environmental
  organization has been promoting

research, education and solutions
particularly in the area of air and water
quality.

Ontario Ministry of the
   Environment
Air Quality Index Reports online:
www.airqualityontario.com

Toronto Enviromental Alliance
30 Duncan Street, Suite 201
Toronto, Ontario M5V 2C3
416-596-0660
Fax: 416-596-0345
www.torontoenvironment.org
• Provides an activist voice to local
  Toronto issues. Main interests are smog
  and climate change, urban pesticides,
  waste reduction, sustainable transportation, water. Newsletter.

Women's Healthy Environments
   Network
24 Mercer Street, Suite 101
Toronto, Ontario M5V 1H3
416-928-0880
Fax: 416-928-9640
Email: **when@web.ca**
www.web.net/~when
• Educates media, policy makers and
  general public on environmentally linked
  health problems. Promotes prevention.
  Video **Exposure: Environment Links to
  Breast Cancer (1997)** available from
  their website.

Household Hazardous Waste
   Hotline—416-392-4330
*Your Guide to Hazardous Waste in
the Home* published by Works and
Emergency Services Support Services
Metro Hall, Station 1180,
55 John Street, 19th Floor
Toronto, Ontario M5V 3C6

Greenpeace Canada
250 Dundas St. W, Suite 605,
Toronto, ON M5T 2Z5
Phone: 416-597-8408
1-800-320-7183
Fax: 416-597-8422
www.greenpeace.ca
• Greenpeace has put out a shoppers'
  guide to food containing genetically
  engineered ingredients on grocery
  shelves. Available from the 1-800 number
  or follow link on website.

Greenpeace International
www.greenpeace.org

Sierra Club—Eastern Canada
   Chapter
24 Mercer Street
Toronto, Ontario, M5V 1H3
416-960-9606
Fax: 416-960-0020
www.sierraclub.ca/eastern
• Publishes newsletter, *Sanctuary*, with
  membership

Sierra Club of Canada
www.sierraclub.ca
• Deals with issues ranging from climate
  change and energy to toxic chemical
  contamination and loss of biological
  diversity working on matters of public
  policy and environmental awareness.
  Extensive information available on
  website.

Sierra Club (US)
www.sierraclub.org

World Wildlife Fund Canada
245 Eglinton Ave. East, Suite 410
Toronto, ON M4P 3J1
416-489-8800
1-800-26-PANDA
Fax: 416-489-8055
www.wwfcanada.org
• Offers several publications with information on pesticides, persistent organic
  pollutants (POPs) and hormone disrupting
  chemicals. Order by phone or follow link
  from website.

World Wildlife Fund International
www.panda.org
• WWF has launched a global campaign to
  reduce the use of toxic chemicals. Follow
  the link to "Toxics" for information,
  publications, research, etc.

RESOURCES

Linus Pauling Institute
Oregon State University
571 Weniger Hall
Corvallis, OR 97331-6512
phone: 541-737-5075
fax: 541-737-5077
www.orst.edu/dept/lpi
• Information on the function and role of micronutrients, phytochemicals, and microconstituents of food in maintaining human health and preventing and treating disease.

National Institute of Environmental
    Health Sciences
Office of Communications
P.O. Box 12233, MD NH-10
Research Triangle Park,
North Carolina 27709-2233
http://www.niehs.nih.gov/
• One of the National Institutes of Health, its website offers research information and the journal **Environmental Health Perspectives** online

McGill University, Montreal,
    Quebec:
Faculty of Agriculture and
Environmental Science:
Ecological Agriculture:
http://www.agrenv.mcgill.ca/
agrecon/ecoagr/

Ecological Agricultural Projects at
    McGill University
http://www.eap.mcgill.ca/
• Both websites are excellent and have extensive information on organic and sustainable agriculture, organic gardening, pest control, etc. for both academics and the lay person.

www.ourstolenfuture.org
• This is the web home for the authors of **Our Stolen Future**. Dr. Theo Colborn, lead author, is a senior scientist with the World Wildlife Fund-US and one of the world's leading authorities on endocrine disrupting chemicals in the environment. She received her Ph.D. in zoology from the University of Wisconsin at Madison and speaks regularly to scientific groups, health officials and policy makers.
• The website provides regular updates about the emerging science related to endocrine disruption, challenging the basic assumptions about which chemicals are safe and what exposures are tolerable. They also post information about ongoing policy debates, as well as new suggestions about what you can do as a consumer and citizen to minimize risks related to hormonally-disruptive contaminants.

RESOURCES

Environmental Working Group
Headquarters 1436 U St. N.W.,
Suite 100, Washington, DC 20009
(202) 667-6982 |
www.ewg.org
• EWG specializes in providing useful
resources (like *Skin Deep* and the *Shoppers' Guide to Pesticides in Produce*) to
consumers while simultaneously pushing
for national policy change.

SUPPLIERS AND SERVICES

Healthy Home Services Inc.
613-623-0933
1-800-819-1598
Fax: 613-623-0910
www.healthyhomeservices.ca
• Fragrance-free and dye-free products,
chemical-free lawn and garden programs

Healthy Home
2894 22nd Ave N
Saint Petersburg, FL 33713
www.healthyhome.com
• Online store for non-toxic products

Needs—Nutritional, Ecological &
Environmental Delivery System
P.O. Box 580
East Syracuse, N.Y. 13057
(800) 634-1380
Fax: (800) 295-NEED
E-mail: **needs@needs.com**
www.needs.com

• Products for the environmentally
sensitive

American Environmental Health
Foundation
(214) 361-9515
Fax: 214-361-2534
1-800-428-2343
E-mail: **aehf@aehf.com**
www.aehf.com
• Associated with the Environmental
Health Center-Dallas offers information
and products for the environmentally
sensitive

Sleeptek Manufacturer of Bedding
and Accessories
50 Colonnade Rd., Ottawa, ON
613.727.5337
Fax. 613.727.1857
E-mail: **info@sleeptek.ca**
http://www.sleeptek.ca
• Organic Mattresses & Pillows
• Natural latex mattresses

The Original Bug Shirt Company
Box 127
Trout Creek, Ontario P0H 2L0
(705) 729-5620
1-800-998-9096
www.bugshirt.com

SAMINA Canada
Natural By Design
Herrn Claus Pummer
276 Carlaw Avenue #9

RESOURCES

Port Carling, ON P0B 1J0
705-765-1882
Fax: 705-765-1884
www.pummer.com
www.samina.com
• Organic beds and bedding products

Small & Rubin LTD.
Bruce M. Small, P.Eng., Director,
Envirodesic™ Certification Program
Research Office, 100 Rexway Drive
Georgetown, Ontario L7G 1R5
Tel: 905-702-8615
Fax: 905-873-6260
E-mail: **enquire@envirodesic.com**
www.envirodesic.com
• Consultation on Indoor Air Quality
  products and services;
• *Envirodesic*™ Certification Program

Quorum Allergy Care
A Division of Quorum Holdings Inc.
Calgary, AB
Toll free tel: 1-866-551-0142
www.quorumallergy.com

Healthy Body Now
Clean Drinking Water & Indoor Air
47-646 Village Pkwy.
Markham, ON, L3R 2S7
905-470-2259

High Tech Health
4888 Pearl East Circle, Suite 202W
Boulder, CO 80301 U.S.A.
1-800-794-5355
www.hightechhealth.com
• Makers of far infrared home saunas
  made from poplar wood

Ed Lowans
425 Echo Drive,
Ottawa, Ontario, KL1S 1N6,
613-237-6302,
Email: **edlowans@rogers.com**
• Assess problem buildings and help specify
  healthy and environmentally appropriate
  materials and design elements for new
  ones. Many years of experience with
  environmental hypersensitivity.

Andrew Michrowski (d.Arch),
    President
The Planetary Association for
Clean Energy, Inc.
100 Bronson Avenue, Suite 1001
Ottawa, Ontario K1R 6G8
(613) 236-6265
Fax: (613) 235-5876
E-mail: **pacenet@canada.com**
www.pacenet.homestead.com
• Assessment of electromagnetic field
  radiation.
• Recommends the following competent
  resource electricians to trace and fix
  miswiring and other electromagnetic
  problems cross-Canada:

Chris Anderson Associates: professional assessment and mitigation of electro-magnetic radiation—to Building Biology standards Tel: 250-537-5102
Walter McGinnis: "Electromagnetic Solutions" – low EMR-wiring for Healthy Homes Tel: 250-652-2554
Nichol Mowat (204) 885-2888
Jean-Claude Morin (819) 868-6643

Breathing Easy—Environmental
   Analysis and Technology
Robert Steller
4 Louisa Street East
P.O. Box 775
Thornbury, Ontario N0H 2P0
Phone / Fax (519) 599–1111
E-mail: info@breathing-easy.net
www.breathing-easy.net
• Products & Services for Healthy Buildings
• Indoor Air Quality, Mould and Microbial Assessments
• Chemical off gassing
• Mould and water damage remediation
• Electromagnetic exposure and microwave assessments
• Assessment of exposure to wireless technology

Medi-Air Inc/TiBBiTS
1200 Fewster Drive,
Mississauga, Ontario L4W 1A1
905-625-8884 Fax: 905-625-4848
www.medi-air.com

www.tibbitsair.com
• Air purification for people with Environ-mental Sensitivities

Haverkate & Associates Inc.
4936 Yonge Street, Suite 191
Toronto, ON M2N 6S3
905-882-2202
www.indoormold.ca
• Indoor Environmental Testing and Consulting

Sick Building Solutions
204 Brown's Line,
Etobicoke, ON, M8W 3T4
416-259-8833 or 1-877-SICKBLD
www.sickbuildingsolutions.com
• Indoor Air Quality Specialists, Mould Inspection and Remediation

Breathe Architects Inc.
Martin Liefhebber + Associates
177 First Avenue
Toronto, Ontario M4M 1X3
416-469-0018
Fax: 416-469-0987
E-mail:
info@breathebyassociation.com
www.breathebyassociation.com
• Affordable and green building design and construction

RESOURCES

SUPPORTIVE RESOURCES FOR ENVIRONMENTALLY SENSITIVE PATIENTS

Human Ecology Action League
    (HEAL)
P.O. Box 29629
Atlanta, GA 30359-0629
(404) 248-1898
Fax: (404) 248-0162
E-mail: **HEALNatnl@aol.com**
**www.members.aol.com/
    HEALNatnl**

Environmental Illness Society of
    Canada (EISC)
536 Dovercourt Avenue
Ottawa, Ontario K2A 0T9
(613) 728-9493
E-mail: **eisc@eisc.ca**
www.eisc.ca

National Me/FM Action Network
3836 Carling Ave.
Nepean, ON K2K 2Y5
Phone/Fax: (613) 829-6667
www.mefmaction.net
• A clearing house for information on
  Myalgic Encephalomyelitis/Chronic
  Fatigue Syndrome and Fibromyalgia.

Nova Scotia Allergy and Environ-
    mental Health Association
P.O. Box 31323
Halifax, Nova Scotia B3K 5Y5
1-800-449-1995
www.environmentalhealth.ca

Total Wellness
Dr. Sherry Rogers' monthly newsletter
Prestige Publishing, P.O. Box 3068
Syracuse, NY, 13220
1-800-846-6687
www.prestigepublishing.com

ALTERNATIVE CANCER TREATMENT RESOURCES

National Foundation for
    Alternative Medicine
5 Thomas Circle NW, Suite 500
Washington, DC 20005
202-463-4900
Fax: 202-463-4947
E-mail: **info@nfam.org**
www.nfam.org
• A global resource center, its mission is
  to review effective complementary and
  alternative medical treatments. Offers
  comprehensive information on alternative
  cancer clinics worldwide.

Cancer Decisions
PO Box 1076
Lemont, PA, 16851
Toll Free: 1-800-980-1234
Fax: (814) 238-5865
www.cancerdecisions.com
• Dr. Ralph Moss' Cancer treatment
  information and referral service.
• See also his book in Cancer references
  at the back of this book

RESOURCES

The Breast Cancer Fund
1388 Sutter Street, Suite 400
San Francisco, CA 94109-5400
415-346-8223
Fax: 415-346-2975
E-mail: **info@breastcancerfund.org**
www.breastcancerfund.org
• Focuses on environmental causes of
  breast cancer. Excellent website.

PROFESSIONAL ORGANIZATIONS
Conferences and Training for doctors
Doctor referral for your geographical area

American Academy of
    Environmental Medicine
6505 E. Central Avenue, #296
Wichita, KS 67206
(316) 684-5500 Fax: (316) 684-5709
Email: **administrator@aaemonline.org**
www.aaem.com

American College for Advancement
    in Medicine
24411 Ridge Route, Ste 115
Laguna Hills, CA 92653
949.309.3520
Fax: 949.309.3538
E-mail: **info@acam.org**
www.acam.org

Pan American Allergy Society
P.O. Box 700587
San Antonio, Texas 78270-0587

210-495-9853
Fax: 210-495-9852
E-mail: **panamallergy@sbcglobal.net**
www.paas.org

American Holistic Medical
    Association
PO Box 2016, Edmonds, WA 98020
425-967-0737
Fax: 425-771-9588
www.holisticmedicine.org

International Society For
    Orthomolecular Medicine
16 Florence Ave
Toronto, Ontario M2N 1E9
416-733-2117
Fax: 416-733-2352
www.orthomed.org

Canadian Complementary Medical
    Association
www.ccmadoctors.ca

Canadian Society for Environmen-
    tal Medicine
3364 Carling Avenue
Ottawa, ON K2H 5A8
www.eimed.ca

Ontario Society of Physicians for
    Complementary Medicine
600 Sherbourne Street, Suite 207
Toronto, Ontario M4X 1W4
www.ospcm.org

RESOURCES

Environmental Health Clinic
Women's College Hospital—
Main Building, 76 Grenville Street,
5th Floor, Room 538 (west wing)
Toronto, ON M5S 1B2
416-351-3764
Toll Free: 1-800-417-7092
Fax: 416-323-6130
www.womenscollegehospital.ca

Nova Scotia Environmental
    Health Centre
3064 Lake Thomas Drive
Fall River, NS, B2T 1K6
(902) 860-3066 Fax: (902) 860-2046
E-mail: **gail.sedgwick@cdha.nshealth.ca**

Canadian College of Naturopathic
    Medicine (CCNM)
1255 Sheppard Ave East
Toronto, Ontario M2K 1E2
416-498-1255   1-866-241-2266
www.ccnm.edu

LABORATORIES

Accu-Chem Laboratories
990 North Bowser, Suite 800
Richardson, Texas 75081
972-234-5412
(800) 451-0116
Fax: 972-234-5707
www.accuchem.com

Doctor's Data, Inc.
3755 Illinois Avenue,
St. Charles, IL USA 60174-2420
Toll free: 1.800.323.2784
630-377-8139
Fax: 630-587-7860
E-mail: **inquiries@doctorsdata.com**
www.doctorsdata.com

Anderson Laboratories
6330 Industrial Loop
Greendale, WI 53129
1-800-950-6330
E-mail: **sales@andersonlabs.com**
www.andersonlabs.com

BodyBio Inc.
Customer Service
45 Reese Road, Millville, NJ
08332, USA
1-888-320-8338 or 856-825-8338
Fax: 856-825-2143

Bowen Research and
    Training Institute
Lake Alfred
245 North Seminole Avenue,
Lake Alfred, Florida 33850
Phone: 863.956.3538
www.bowen.org

The Great Plains Laboratory
11813 W. 77th Street
Lenexa, KS 66214

(913) 341-8949
Fax: (913) 341-6207
www.greatplainslaboratory.com

Genova Diagnostics
63 Zillicoa Street
Asheville, NC 28801, USA
828-253-0621
www.gdx.net

Nutrichem Biomedical Laboratory
1303 Richmond Rd, Suite 205
Ottawa, ON
(613) 820-6755
Fax: (613) 820-6985
www.nutrichem.com

Immunosciences Lab., Inc.
8693 Wilshire Blvd., Suite 200
Beverly Hills, CA 90211
(310) 657-1077
Fax: (310) 657-1053
Toll Free: (800) 950-4686
www.immunoscienceslab.com

London Health Sciences Centre
Department of Laboratory Medicine
Trace Elements Lab, University Campus
P.O. Box 5339, Windermere Rd.,
London, Ontario N6A 5A5

Metametrix Clinical Laboratory
3425 Corporate Way
Duluth, GA 30096
770-446-5483 or 1-800-221-4640
Fax: 770-441-2237

York Nutritional Laboratory,
Murton Way, Osbaldwick, York
YO19 5US   United Kingdom
+44 (0) 1904 410410
Fax: +44 (0) 01904 422000
E-mail: **ynl@allergy-testing.com**
www.allergy-testing.com
ILADS — International Lyme and
Associated Disease Society
P.O. Box 341461 Bethesda, MD
20827-1461
www.ilads.org

Igenex Inc. Reference Laboratory
795 San Antonio Rd.
Palo Alto, CA 94303
(800) 832-3200
Fax: (650) 424-1196
E-mail: **Igenex@igenex.com**
www.igenex.com

Medical Diagnostic Laboratory L.L.C.
2439 Kuser Rd, Hamilton, NJ 08690
609 570 1000
Fax: 609 570 1050
E-mail: **info@mdlab.com**
www.mdlab.com

Laboratoire Philippe Auguste
119 Philippe Auguste
7501 Paris, France
(33) 1 43 67 57 00
Fax: (33) 1 43 79 00 27
Email: **contact@labbio.net**
http://www.labbio.net

RESOURCES

COMPOUNDING HOLISTIC PHARMACIES

Abrams Royal Pharmacy
8220 Abrams Road
Dallas, Texas
(214) 349-8000
www.abramsroyalpharmacy.com

Hooper's Pharmacy
88 Lakeshore Road East,
Mississauga L5G 1E1
905.278.4242
Toll Free: 1.800.201.2813
Fax: 905.278.9468
Email: **pc@hoopershealth.com**
www.hoopershealth.com

Tecumseh Big V Drug Store
1125 Lesperance Road
Tecumseh, Ontario
(519) 735-2121

Glebe Pharmasave Apothecary
778 Bank Street, Ottawa, Ontario
(613) 234-8587
www.apothecary.on.ca

Atrium Pharmacy
190 Cundles Road
Barrie, Ontario
(705) 734-2121

The Medicine Shoppe
10610 Bayview Ave.

Richmondhill ,ON
905-884-2866
Fax: 905-844-5453

Port Credit Village Pharmacy
225 Lakeshore Road East
Mississauga, Ontario
905-278-7237

Smith's Pharmacy
3463 Yonge Street
Toronto, Ontario M4N 2N3
416-488-2600
Fax: 416-484-8855
Toll Free: 1-800-361-6624
www.smithspharmacy.com

York Downs Pharmacy
3910 Bathurst Street
North York, Ontario
416-633-2244
1-800-564-5020
www.yorkdownsrx.com

Canadian Apothecary
1064 Adelaide St. North
London, Ontario
(519) 439-4100

Kripps Pharmacy Ltd.
994 Granville Street
Vancouver, B.C.
(604) 687-2564
Fax: (604) 685-9721
www.krippspharmacy.com

Central Medical Pharmacy
311 Sherbourne Street
Toronto, Ontario
416-960-7768
www.pharmacy.ca

Nutricam Pharmacy
1303 Richmond Road
Ottawa, Ontario
(613) 820-9065

The Wellness Pharmacy
420 Erb Street
Waterloo, Ontario
(519) 884-1025

Hunters Pharmacy
3019 Tecumseh Road E
Windsor, Ontario
(519) 945-4333

Health Care Pharmacy
1276 La Salle Blvd.
Sudbury, Ontario
(705) 566-5551

Guardian Pharmacy
15017 Yonge St. #204
Aurora, ON
905-727-1343
Fax: 905-727-0845

The Medicine Shoppe
2917 Bloor St. W.
Toronto, ON
416-239-3566

Dell Pharmacy
Main Street
Beamsville, ON
905-563-8196

Hill Ave Drugs Ltd.
Regina, Saskatchewan
306-586-6262
Fax: 306-584-7948

The Medicine Shoppe
Sault Ste. Marie, ON
705-253-0720
Fax:705-253-7656

The Medicine Shoppe
Peterborough — 705-743-9443
Whitby — 905-7218676

Medical Arts Pharmacy
Saskatoon City
306-652-5252

IDA
603 Clarkson Rd. N.
Mississauga, ON
905-823-4664

Plaza 69 Pharmacy
1935 Paris St. Sudbury, ON
705-522-2121

Pharmasave
101–45 Wyndham St. N.
Guelph, ON
519-763-0695 Fax: 519-763-9792

RESOURCES

Women's International Pharmacy
1-800-279-5708
Fax:1-800-279-8011

Brant Arts Dispenserary
672 Brant St.
Burlington, ON
905-637-3833 1-866-939-0002
www.brantarts.com

Guardian Pharmacy
400 Laclie St., Orilia, ON
705-325-1111
Fax: 705-325-8644

River Run Pharmasave
1525 Bristol Rd. W.
Mississauga,ON L5M 4Z1
905-819-1999
Fax: 905-819-8692

RESOURCES

Bibliography

PRINCIPLES OF ENVIRONMENTAL MEDICINE

Bell, Iris R. *Clinical Ecology: A New Medical Approach To Environmental Illness*, Common Courage Press, 1982

Cullen, Mark R. *Workers with Multiple Chemical Sensitivities*, Hanley and Belfus Inc., Philadelphia, Vol. 2, No.4 Oct–Dec, 1987

Cunningham, Alastair J., *Mind, Body and Immune Response, Psychoneuro-Immunology*, Edited by Robert Ader, Academic Press, Inc., 1981

Dickey, Lawrence, ed. *Clinical Ecology*, Springfield, Illinois, Charles C. Thomas, 1976

Miller, J.B. *Food Allergy: Provocative Testing and Injection Therapy*, Charles. C. Thomas, 1972

O'Banion, D.R. *Ecological and Nutritional Treatment of Health Disorder*, Charles C. Thomas, 1981.

Randolph, Theron G. and Moss, Ralph, W. *An Alternative Approach to Allergies*, Lippincott & Crowell Publishing, N. Y.

Randolph, Theron G. *Environmental Medicine—Beginnings and Bibliographies of Clinical Ecology*, Citizen Printing, Fort Collins, Colorado, 1987

Rea, William. *Chemical Sensitivity Volume (Vol 1-4)*, Lewis Publishers 1994

Rinkel, H, Randolph, T, Zeller. R *Food Allergy*, Charles C. Thomas, 1951

Rogers, S. *The Scientific Basis for Selected Environmental Medicine Techniques*, SK Publishers, 1994

Werbach, R.M. *Nutritional Influences on Mental Illness*, Third Line Press, 1999

Multiple Chemical Sensitivity: A 1999 Consensus. *Archives of Environmental Medicine*. May/June, 1999 Vol 54, No. 3.

Safety of Immunotherapy

Cook, PR et al. Systemic reactions to Immunotherapy: The AAOA Morbidity and Mortality Survey. *Otolaryngol Head Neck Surg* 1993.

Lockey, RF et al. Fatalities from immunotherapy (IT) and skin testing (ST). *J.Allergy Clin Immunol*. Vol 79, No.4, April 1987, pp 660-677

Reid, MF et al. Survey of fatalities from skin testing and immunotherapy 1985-1989. *J Allergy Clinn Immunol*. Vol. 92, No. 1, Part 1, July 1993, pp 6-15.

Reid, MJ et al. Fatalities from immunotherapy (IT) 1990-91. *J Allergy Clin Immunol* 1992; 89:350.

Stewart, GE. Systemic reactions from allergen immunotherapy. Editorial in *J Allergy Clin Immunol*, Vol 90, No. 4, Part 1, October 1992, pp 567-578

Report of a British Society of Allergy and Clinical Immunology (BSACI) Working Party. Position Paper on Allergen Immunotherapy. *Clinical and Experimental Allergy*, Vol 23, Supp 3, August 1993.

Autogenous Vaccine

Kasckin, PN. Some Aspects of the Candidiasis Problem. *Mycopathologia et Mycologia applicata,* Vol 53, pp 173-181, 1974.

Livi, U et al. The use of an autogenous vaccine in the treatment of sternal wound infections following open heart procedures: a preliminary report. *Ital J Surg Sci.* 14(1): 17-20, 1984.

Okrasinska-Cholewa, B. Assessment of Clinical treatment of sinus infections in children with autovaccines. *Med Dosw Mikrobiol,* 1994, 46, S 67-73

Rea, Wm. *Chemical Sensitivity,* Vol. 1V, pp 2520-2522 Lewis Publishers, Boca Raton, 1997 .

Wiltz, OH et al. Autogenous Vaccine: The best therapy for perianal condyloma acuminata? *Dis Colon Rectum,* August 1995, pp 838-841

Electrodermal Testing

Ali, Majid. Correlation of IgE Antibodies with specificity for pollen and mold allergy with changes in electrodermal skin responses following exposure to allergens. Abstract. *Am J Pathology* 1989: 91(3): 357.

Fox, A. Determination of neutralisation point for allergic hypersensitivity. *British Homeopathic Journal,* 1987; 76: 230-234.

Krop, J et al. Comparison of Ecological Testing with the Vega Test Method in Identifying Sensitivities to Chemicals, Foods and Inhalants. *Am J Acupuncture,* 1985; 13(3): 253-260.

Krop, J et al. A Double blind, randomised, controlled investigation of electrodermal testing in the diagnosis of allergies. *J Alternative and Complementary Medicine,* Vol 3, No. 3, 1997, pp 241-248.

Krop, J et al. A double blind comparison of electrodermal testing with serial dilution end-point titration and skin prick tests for allergy to house dust mite. *Am J of Acupuncture,* Vol 26, No. 1, 1998, pp 53-62.

Royal, FF et al. A review of the history and scientific bases of electrodiagnosis and it relationship to homeopathy and acupuncture. *Am J Acupuncture,* 1991: 19(2):137-152.

Tiller, WA. On the evolution and future development of electrodermal diagnostic instruments. In: *Energy Fields in Medicine: A study of device technology based on acupuncture meridians and CHI energy.* John E. Fetzer Foundation, Kalamazoo, Mich. 1989: 257-328.

Tiller, WA. Explanation of electrodermal diagnostic and treatment instruments: Part I. Electrical behaviour of human skin. *Journal of Holistic Medicine,* 1982, 4(2): 105-127.

Tsuie, JJ et al. A Food Allergy Study Utilizing the EAV Acupuncture Technique. *Am J Acupuncture,* Vol 12, No 2, April-June 1984

American Association of Acupuncture and Bioenergetic Medicine 2512 Manoa Road, Honolulu, HI 96822 *www.aaabem.org*

INHALANTS, FUNGI, MOLDS

Barkowski, DP et al. Emphysematous prostatitis and cystitis secondary to Candida albicans. *J Urol* 1988:139(5): 1063-5.

Bodey, GP. ed. *Candidiasis: Pathogenesis, Diagnosis and Treatments.* Raven Press, 1993

Cantani A. et al. Recent advances in Candida albicans mycoses in children. *Riv Eur Sci Med Farmacol* 1989;11(1):17-20.

Cohen, SR, Thompson JW. Otitic candidiasis in children: an evaluation of the problem and effectiveness of ketoconazole in 10 patients. *Ann Otol Rhinol Laryngol* 1990; 99(6): 427-31.

Crook, WG. *The Yeast Connection* Vintage Books, 1986

Crook, WG. *Dr. Crook Discusses Yeasts and How They Can Make You Sick* Tennessee, Professional Books, 1984

Edwards DA. Depression and Candida. *JAMA* 1985; 253(23):3400.

Gates, D., *The Body Ecology Diet,* 6th ed. B.E.D. Publishers, 1998

Hollister-Stier Division of Cutter Laboratories, Inc. *Plants of Allergic Importance 1979*

Gershon, MD. *The Second Brain: Your Gut Has A Mind Of Its Own,* Harper Collins, 1998

Gotlieb JK, Andersen J. Occurrence of candida in gastric ulcers. Significance for the healing Process. Gastroenterology (US) 1983; 85/3:535-37.

Hernanadez, YL, Daniels TE. Oral candidiasis in Sjorgren's syndrome: prevalence, clinical correlation and treatment. *Oral Surg Oral Med Oral Pathol* 1989; 68(2): 188-93.

Kligman AM. Are fungus infections increasing as a result of antibiotic therapy? *JAMA* July 12, 1952; 149: 979-83.

Liebeskind A. Candida albicans as an allergenic factor. *Ann Allergy* 1962; 20: 394-96.

Morris, AB. et al. Gallbladder and biliary tract candidiasis: nine cases and review. *Rev Infect Dis* 1990;12(3):484-9.

Truss, CO. *The Missing Diagnosis*. Birmingham, AL. Missing Diagnosis, Inc. 1982.

Trowbridge, JP, Walker M. *The Yeast Syndrome*. Bantam Books, NY 1986.

CHEMICALS

Ashford, Nicholas and Miller, Claudia, S. *Chemical Exposures—Low Levels and High Stakes 2nd edition*, Van Nostrand Reinhold, N.Y., 1998

Ashley, DL. et al. Blood concentrations of volatile organic compounds I a non-occupationally exposed US population and in groups with suspected exposure. *Clin Biochem* 1994; 40/7:1401-1404.

Brown, M. *Laying Waste: The Poisoning of America by Toxic Chemicals*, Pantheon Books, 1980.

Brown, M. *The Toxic Cloud: The Poisoning of America's Air.* Harper Row, 1987.

Chivion, Eric, *Critical Condition: Human Health and the Environment*, MIT Press, Cambridge, Mass. 1994.

Cone, James and Hodgson, Michael. *Problem Buildings—Building, Associated Illness and the Sick Building Syndrome*, Vol. 4, No. 4, Oct.–Dec. 1989, Hanley & Belfus, Inc. Philadelphia

Fagin, D. & Lavelle, M. *Toxic Deception*, Common Courage Press, 1999

Kilburn, K.H. *Chemical Brain Injury*, Van Nostrand Reinhold, 1998

Klaassen, Curtis, Amdur, Mary, and Doull, John. *Casarett & Doull's Toxicology: The Basic Science of Poisons*, MacMillan Publishing Co., 1986

Kosta, Louise A. *Fragrance and Health*, HEAL, 1998.

Penney, David G., *Carbon Monoxide Toxicity*, CRC Press, Boca Raton FL, June 2000.

Pfeiffer, Guy and Csmkir, Nikel. *The Household Environment and Chronic Illness* Charles C. Thomas, 1980

Wargo, J. *Our Children's Toxic Legacy*, Yale University Press, 1998

Wolff, M. Equilibrium of polybromiated biphenyls (PBB) residue in serum and fats of Michigan residents. Bull Environmental Contamination. *Toxicol* 1979; 21(6); 775-781.

Zussman, B. Tobacco Sensitivity in the Allergic Population, *Journal of Asthma Research* 11; 4: 1974

References specific to UV Light and plants:

Klironomos JN, Allen MF. UVB mediated changes on below-ground communities associated with roots of sugar maples. *Functional Ecology* 1995, 9: 923-930

Manning WJ, Vontiedemann A. 1995 Climate Change—potential effects of increased atmospheric carbon-dioxide (CO_2), ozone (O-3), and ultraviolet-B (UVB) radiation on plant-diseases. *Environmental Pollution* 88:219-245.

Shafer SR, Schoeneberger MM. Mycorrhizal mediation of plant response to atmospheric change—air quality concepts and research considerations. *Environmental Pollution*. 73 (3-4):163-177.

Smith, Cameron. The *Toronto Star* August 17, 2002

Sylvia D et al. Principles and Applications of Soil Microbiology. Prentice Hall 1997.
. Zaller JG et al. Solar UV-B radiation affects below-ground parameters in a fen ecosystem in Tierra del Fuego, Argentina: implications of stratospheric ozone depletion. Global Change Biology 8(9): 867-871

FOOD AND NUTRITION

Batterham, RL et al. Gut hormone PYY 3-36 physiologically inhibits food intake. *Nature,* Vo. 418, Aug. 8, 2002, pp 650-653.

Brostoff, J. and Gamlin. Linda *Food Allergy and Intolerance* Bloomsbery Publ., 1989

Buchholz, ID, Cook, SK, Randolph, TG. *An Alternative Measure,* Human Ecology Research Foundation, 505 North Lakeshore Drive, Chicago, Illinois, USA 60611

Crook, W. *Tracking Down Hidden Food Allergies,* Jackson, Tennessee, Professional Books, 1980

Dufty, W., *Sugar Blues,* Warner Books, 1975

Erasmus, U. *Fats that Heal—Fats that Kill,* Alive Books Canada, 1993

Fletcher, RH and Fairfield, KM, Vitamins for Chronic Disease Prrevention in Adults: Clinical Applictions, *JAMA* 2002;287:3127-3129

Gursche, Siegfried. *Good Fats and Oils,* Alive Books Canada, 2000

Hoffer, A. *Dr. Hoffer's ABC of Natural Nutrition for Children,* Quarry Press, 1999

Hoffer, A. *Hoffer's Laws of Natural Nutrition,* Quarry, 2001

Klee, WA et al. Endorphins in Mental Health Research Conference. Puerto Rico, 1997, pp 209-218.

Lichtenstein, et al. Effects of different forms of dietary hydrogenated fats on serum lipoprotein cholesterol levels. *N Engl J Med* 1999;340:1933-1940, June 24, 1999

Lieberman, S. & Bruning, N. *The Real Vitamin and Mineral Book: Going Beyond the RDA for Optimum Health,* Avery, 1990

` Michels K, Sacks F. Trans fatty acids in Euroean maragarines. *N Engl J Med* 1995;332:541-542, Feb 23, 1995

Miller, JB. Annals of Allergy *"Hidden Food Ingredients, Chemical Food Additives and Incomplete Food Labels"* Vol. 41, No. 2, August 1978

Murray, M T. *Encyclopedia of Nutritional Supplements,* Prima Publ., 1996

Nestle, M. *Food Politics: How the Food Industry Influences Nutrition and Health,* University of California Press, 2002

Peet, Glen & Horrobin, D. *Phospholipid Spectrum Disorder in Psychiatry,* Marius, U.K. 1999

Price, W.A. *Nutrition and Physical Degeneration,* 50th anniversary ed., Keats, 1989

Oski, Frank A. *Don't Drink Your Milk: New Frightening Facts about the World's Most Overrated Nutrient,* Mollica Press, 1983

Roberts, HJ. *Aspartame—Is It Safe?* Charles Press, 1990

Roberts, HJ. *The Aspartame Disease—An Ignored Epidemic,* Sunshine Sentinel Press Inc., 2001

Sapeika N, *Food Pharmacology,* Charles C. Thomas 1969

Sarjeant, D. and Evans, K. *Hard To Swallow: The Truth About Food Additives,* Alive Books Canada, 1999

Pollution Probe Foundation. *Additive Alert!* McClelland & Stewart 1995

Virlanen, S.M. et al. Cow's milk consumption, disease associated antibodies and Type I diabetes milletus: a follow-up study in siblings of diabetic children. *Diabetic Medicine,* vol. 15, 1998

Walter P. et al, Eds. Function of Vitamins beyond Recommended Dietary Allowances, in *Biblioteca Nutritio et Dieta.* No. 55, 2001, S. Karger Publishers

Walter, P. et al, Eds. Role of Trace Elements for Health Promotion and Disease Prevention, in *Biblioteca Nutritio et Dieta,* No. 54, 1998, S. Karger Publishers

Wardlaw, Gordon, Insel, Paul. *Perspectives In Nutrition* Toronto, Times Mirror/Mosby College Publishing, 1990

Werbach, R.M., *Textbook of Nutritional Medicine*, Third Line Press, 1999

Worthington, V. Effect of agricultural methods on nutritional quality: A comparison of organic with conventional crops. *Alternative Therapies in Health and Medicine* 1998; Vol 4, No. 1.

Worthington, V. Nutrition and Biodynamics: Evidence for the nutritional superiority of organic crops. *Biodynamics*, vol 224, Jul/Aug 99.

Tina Finesilver in collaboration with Prof. Timothy Johns and Prof. Stuart B. Hill. Comparison of food quality of organically versus conventionally grown plant foods. *1989 Report is based on a review of literature on the comparative quality of organically versus conventionally grown food. Copies of the materials reviewed in the study are stored at the Ecological Agriculture Projects office, Macdonald College, McGill University, Montreal Canada. www.eap.mcgill.ca/Publications/EAP38.htm*

References and Resources specific to Genetically Engineered Foods:

Baker BP, et al. Pesticide residues in conventional, IPM-grown and organic foods: Insights from three US data sets. *Food Additives and Contaminants*, Vol 19, No. 5, May 2002, pp 427-446.

Boyens, Ingeborg. *Unnatural Harvest*, Doubleday, 1999

Cummins, R. & Lilliston, B. *Genetically Engineered Food: A Self-Defence Guide for Consumers*, Marlow & Co, 2000

Ho, Mae-Wan. *Genetic Engineering: Dream or Nightmare?*, Continum, 2000

Jack, A. *Imagine a World Without Monarch Butterflies*, One Peaceful World Press, 2000

Kneen, Brewster. *Farmageddon: Food and the Culture of Biotechnology* , New Society Publishers, 1999

Lappee, Marc & Bailey, Britt. *Against the Grain*, Common Courage Press, 1998

Roberts W, MacRae R & Stahlbrand L. *Real Food For A Change*, Random, 1999

Rifkin, Jeremy. *The Biotech Century*, Tarcher/Putnam, 1998

Shiva, Vandana. *Stolen Harvest: The Hijacking of the Global Food Supply*, South End Press 2000

Suzuki, D and Dressel, H. *From Naked Ape to Superspecies*, Stoddart, 1999.

Ewen, S and Pusztai, A. Effects of diets containing genetically modified potatoes expressing *Galanthus nivalis* lectin on rat small intestine. *The Lancet* 354:9187,1353.

Dr. Arpad Pusztai is the only scientist to date who succeeded in publishing, at the request of the British Government, food safety studies on genetically engineered foods. Upon publication of these he was fired from his research post and his research data, computers etc. were confiscated by the University of Edinburgh whose major financial source is Monsanto, the bio-tech company that developed genetically engineered plants. The full story and the research data are found on *http://www.freenetpages.co.uk/hp/a.pusztai/*

Sprinkel, Steven. When the corn hits the fan. In Acres US 18 Sept 1999. A reprint of this article is available at *www.mindfully.org/GE/ge-pre2000.htm*

Some websites that provide up-to-date scientific information on developments as well as hazards pertaining to genetic engineering:

Prof. Ann Clark's website: *www.plant.uoguelph.ca/research/homepages/eclark/*

Canadian Food Inspection Agency for information on biotechnology regulation in Canada: *www.inspection.gc.ca*

The Women's Environmental Network *www.wen.org.uk*

Organic Consumers Association (a global clearinghouse for information and grassroots technical assistance): *www.organicconsumers.org*

BIBLIOGRAPHY

An excellent source on GE is a film made by the National Film Board of Canada in January 2000 entitled *The Genetic Take-Over or Mutant Foods*. Some of the world's experts, including Prof. Pusztai, are interviewed and all the currently documented health risks are clearly explained. (For $20.00 call from the NFB: 1-800-267-7710.)

MANAGEMENT

Bower, John. *The Healthy House*, General Publishing Co., 1989
Chiu, Beverly. *How You Can Outsmart your Food Allergies*, Vancouver, Yellow hat Press, 1987
Cranton, Elmer. *Bypassing Bypass, The New Technique of Chelation Therapy* Hampton Roads Publishing Company, 1992
Dadd, Debra Lynn. Home Safe Home. Tarcher/Putnam, 1997
Dadd, Debra Lynn. *Nontoxic and Natural,* Jeremy P. Tarcher, 1984
Erikson, K., *Drop-Dead Gorgeous: Protecting Yourself from the Hidden Dangers of Cosmetics,* MacGraw Hill, 2002
Faelten, Sharon and Editors of Prevention Magazine, *The Allergy Self Help Book* Emmaus, Pa, Rodale Press, 1983
Frazier, Claude, A., *Coping with Food Allergy,* New York, New York Times Book
Gibson, P.R. *Multiple Chemical Sensitivity: A Survival Guide*, New Harbinger, 2000
Golos, Natalie and Golos Golbitz, Francis *Coping With Your Allergies* New York, Simon and Schuster, 1979
Gorman, Carolyn P. *Less-Toxic Living Sixth Edition.* Environmental Health Centre, Dallas, Texas 1990. Available from NEEDS 1-800-634-1380.
Harris, M., *Ecological Gardening: Your Path to A Healthy Garden*, Random House, 1991
Hurt, Jones, Marjorie, *The Allergy Self Help Cookbook* Emmaus, PA, Rodale Press, 1984
Martin, Jeanne Marie, *All Natural Allergy Recipes: Gluten and Dairy Free* Vancouver, J.M.M. Publications, 1986
Miller, JB. *Relief At Last! Neutralization for Food Allergy and Other Illnesses* Springfield, Illinois, Charles C. Thomas, 1987
Pim, L., *The Invisible Additive: Environmental Contaminants In Our Food* Toronto, Doubleday, 1981
Rousseau, Rea, Enwright, *Your Home, Your Health and Wellbeing* Vancouver, Hartley and Marks Publishing, 1988
Shattuck, Ruth, *The Allergy Cookbook* New York, Penguin Inc., 1984
Spangler, Tina. *The Solution for Indoor Pollution.* Natural Health Jan/Feb 1995 p 42.
Steinman D, Epstein S. *The Safe Shopper's Bible: A consumer's guide to non-toxic household products, cosmetics and food.* MacMillan, N.Y., 1995.
Sullivan, K. *Organic Living: in 10 simple lessons.* Barron's, 2001
The Pollution Probe Foundation, *The Canadian Green Consumer Guide* McClelland & Stewart 1988.
Thrasher, Jack, and Broughton, Alan. *The Poisoning of Our Homes & Workplaces* Copyright 1989 Seadora, Inc.
Too, Lillian. *The Complete Illustrated Guide to Feng Shui* Element Books Ltd. 1996
Weiss, Linda, *The Kitchen Magician: A Substitution Cookbook* Milford, M.I., Prosperity Publishing, 1986
Zamn, AV., and Cannon, R., *Why Your House May Endanger Your Health* N.Y., Simon and Schuster, 1980

SPECIAL INTEREST
ADHD
Breggin, P. *Talking Back To Ritalin*, Common Courage Press, 1998
Crook, WG. *Help for the Hyperactive Child*. Professional Books, Inc., Jackson TN 1991.
Crook, WG. And Stevens, L, *Solving The Puzzle of Your Hard-To-Raise Child* Random House, 1991
Rapp, Doris. *The Impossible Child* Buffalo, N.Y. Practical Allergy Research Foundation, 1986
Rapp, Doris. *Is It Your Child* William Morrow and Co., 1991
Rapp, Doris. *Is This Your Child's World?* Bantam Books, October 1996.

EPD
Astartia C et al. A double-blind placebo-controlled trail of enzyme potentiated desensitization in the treatment of pollenosis. *J Invest Allergol Clin Immunol* (1996); 6(4): 248-255
Cantani A et al. Enzyme potentiated desensitization in children with asthma and mite allergy: A double-blind study. *J Invest Allergol Clin Immunol*, (1996); 6(4): 270-276
Caramia G, et al. The efficacy of EPD, a new immunotherapy, in the treatment of allergic diseases in children. *Allergie et Immunologie* (1996) 28(9); 308-310
Eggar, J, Stolla A, McEwen LM. Controlled trial of hyposensitisation I children with food-induced hyperkinetic syndrome. *Lancet* (1992) 339; 1150-1153
Egger J et al. Controlled trial of hyposensitisation in children with food-induced migraine. *Cephalalgia,* (1993) ; 13 (Suppl 13); 216
Fell, P and Brostoff, J. A single-dose desensitization for summer hay fever: Results of a double-blind study 1988. *Eur J Clin Pharmacol* (1990) 38; 77-79
Galland L, McEwen LM. A role for food intolerance in childhood migraine. *World Ped and Child care* (1996) 6:-2-8
McEwen, LM and Starr, MS. Enzyme potentiated hyposensitisation: The effect of pre-treatment with B-glucuronidase, hyaluronidase and antigen on anaphylactic sensitivity of guinea pigs, ats and mice. *Int Arch Allergy* (1972) 42; 152-158.
McEwen, LM. Enzyme potentiated hyposensitisation V: Five case reports of patients with acute food allergy. *Ann Allergy* (1975) 35; 98-103.
McEwen, LM. A double-blind controlled trial of enzyme potentiated hyposensitsation for the treatment of ulcerative colitis. Clin ecology, (1987) 5;47-51
Pulec JL. Enzyme potentiated desensitization: a major breakthrough (Editorial). *Ear, Nose & Throat Journal* (1996) 75(10); 640

Hydrotherapy (Sauna)
Krop, J. Chemical sensitiviy after intoxication at work with solvents: Response to sauna therapy, *Jour Alt Comp Med 1998*; 4, 1: 77-86
Matej J, Palat M. Sauna rehabilitacia. XVI/1983 Supplement 26-27. VIIIth International Congress on Sauna, Sept. 20-23, 1982
Rea, WJ. Chemical Sensitivity (Vol 4), p 2334-2446. Lewis Publishers, 1997
Roehm DC. Effect of a program of sauna baths and megavitamins on adipose DDE and PCBs and on clearing of symptoms of Agent orange (dioxin) toxicity. *Clin Res* 1983; 31:243
Schnare DW et al. Evaluation of detoxification rgimen for fat store xenobiotics. *Med Hypothesis* 1982; 9:265-282
Tretjak, et al. Occupation, environmental and public health in Semic: A case study of polychlorinated biphenyls (PCB) pollution: Post Audits of Environmental Programs and Projects; New York, N.Y. American Society of Civil Engineers 1989; 57-72

BIBLIOGRAPHY

WHO, Nordic Council of Ministers 1985. Organic solvents and central nervous system, EH5 Copenhagen, Denmark, World Health Organization Nordi Council of Ministers, pp 1-39

Hormones
Berkson, D.L., *Hormone Deception,* Contemporary Books, 2000
Colborn, T., Dumanoski, D. & Myers, J.P., *Our Stolen Future,* Plume Books, 1997
Jefferies, W., *Safe Uses of Cortisone,* Charles Thomas Publ., 1981
Lee, J.R., *What Your Doctor May Not Tell You About Menopause,* Warner Books, 1996
Reiss, U., *Natural Hormone Balance,* Pocket Books, 2001

Stealth Infections
Ewald, PW. *Plague Time: The New Germ Theory of Disease.* Anchor Books, 2002
Tilley, BC et al. Minocycline in Rheumatoid Arthritis, *Annals of Internal Medicine* 1995; 122:81-89

Dental Amalgams
Casdorph, H. & Walker, M., *Toxic Metal Syndrome: How Metal Poisonings Can Affect Your Brain,* Avery, 1995
Hallaway, N. RN & Strauts, Z., MD, *Turning Lead Into Gold: How Heavy Metal Poisoning Can Affect Your Child and How to Prevent and Treat It,* New Star Books, 1995
Huggins, H., DDS, *It's All In Your Head: The Link Between Mercury Amalgam and Illness,* Avery, 1993
Meining, G.E., DDS, *Root Canal Cover-Up,* Bion, 1996
Walker, M., *Elements of Danger: Protecting Yourself Against the Hazards of Modern Dentistry,* Hampton Roads, 2000

Cancer
Caste, L. *Cancer, Poison, Profits and Prevention,* Common Courage Press, 1996
Diamond, W.J. et al. *Cancer Diagnosis: What to do next,* Alternative Medicine, 2000
Diamond, W.J., Cowden, W.L, Goldberg, B. *Alternative Medicine Definitive Guide to Cancer,* Future Medicine Publishing Inc. 1997
Epstein, Samuel S, Steinman D. *The Breast Cancer Prevention Program.* Macmillan 1997
Gerson, C. & Walker, M., *The Gerson Therapy,* Twin Streams, 2001
Gordon, J.S. & Curtin, S., *Comprehensive Cancer Care,* Perseus, 2000
Hardell, L., Eriksson, M., A Case-Control Study of Non-Hodgkin Lymphoma and Exposure to Pesticides,. *Cancer* Vol. 85, No. 6: 1353-1360.
Hoffer, A., *Vitamin C and Cancer: Discovery, Recovery, Controversy,* Quarry, 2000
Lichenstein, P. et al. Environmental and Heritable Facotrs in the Causation of Cancer—Analysses of cohorts of Twins from Sweden, Denmark and Finland, *New England Journal of Medicine,* 343; 2, July 13, 2000
Moss, R.W., *Questioning Chemotherapy,* Equinox Press, 2000
Moss, RW. *Cancer Therapy: The Independent Consumer's Guide to Non-Toxic Treatment and Prevention.* Equinox Press, 1992
Proctor, R.N. *Cancer Wars: How Politics Shapes What We Know and What We Don't Know About Cancer,* Basic Books, 1995
Sherman, J.D. *Life's Delicate Balance: Causes and Prevention of Breast Cancer,* Taylor & Francis, 2000
Steingraber, S. *Living Downstream: An Ecologist Looks at Cancer and the Environment* Addison Wesley, 2nd ed. 1999
Welch H.G., Black W.C., Are deaths within 1 month of cancer-directed surgery attributed to cancer? *J Natl Cancer Inst* Vol 94, No. 14, 1006-70

Everyday Carcinogens: Stopping cancer before it starts. Workshop on Primary Cancer Prevention 1999. McMaster University, Hamilton, Ontario. *www.stopcancer.org*
Taking action for a healthy future: educational resources guide and community handbook for the film Exposure—environmental links to breast cancer. WHNE Connections. Women's Network on Health and the Environment. Issue 14, Fall 1999, 214 Mercer Street, Suite 102, Toronto, ON M5V 1H3 (416) 928-0880. *www.web.net/~when*
Ron Kennedy. Cancer Prevention. Santa Rosa, Ca. *www.medical-library.net/index.html*

Electromagnetic Radiation (EMR)

Becker, R.O. *Cross Currents: The Perils of Electropollution, The Promise of Electromedicine,* Jeremy P Tarcher Inc., 1990
Minder CE, Pfluger DH, Leukemia, brain tumors, and exposure to extremely low frequency electromagnetic fields in Swiss railway employees., *Am J Epidemiol* May 1 2001, 153(9) p825-35
Smith, CW and Best S. *Electromagnetic Man: Health and Hazard in the Electrical Environment,* J.M. Dent & Sons Ltd., 1989

Nuclear Radiation

Bertell, R. Internal bone-seeking radionuclides and monocyte counts. *International Perspectives in Public Health.* Vol. 9, 21-26, 1993.
Bertell, R. Update of the Chernobyl Disaster: A Critical Analysis. *International Journal of Humanitarian Medicine.* In Press, Fall 2002.
Bertell, R. *Planet Earth: The Latest Weapon of War,* Black Rose Books, Montreal 2001. To order call 1-800-565-9523 or through Amazon.com
Bertell, R. *No Immediate Danger: Prognosis for a Radioactive Earth,* Women's Press, Toronto, 1985
Blot, WJ & Miller, RW. Mental retardation following in utero exposure to the atomic bombs of Hiroshima and Nagasaki. *Radiology,* Vol. 106, 1973, 617-619 Radiology, Vol 106, 617-619, 1973.
Bridges, A.B.,. *Radiation Research,* vol. 156, 631-641, 2001
Burlakova, EB(ED). *Consequences of the Chernobyl Catastrophe: Human Health* (English version), Pensoft Publishers, Moscow 1996.
Nussbaum, R.H., The Linear no-threshold dose-effect relation: Is it relevant to radiation protection regulation. *Medical Physics,* Vol 25, 3, 1998
Nussbaum, R.H. & Kohnlein, W. Inconsistencies and Open Questions Regarding Low-Dose Health Effects of Ionizing Radiation. *Environmental Health Perspectives,* Vol. 102, No. 8, August 1994.
Stewart, A. Malignant Diseases in Childhood and Diagnostic Irradiation in Utero. *The Lancet 1956,* Sept. p 447
Stewart, A. Childhood Cancers in the U.K. and their relations to Background Radiation. *Radiation and Health,* 1987, Vol 16, 201-220.
Zhou, H. et al. Radiation risk to low fluences of a particles may be greater than we thought. *Proceedings of the American Academy of Sciences,* Vol 98, Issue 25, 14410-14415, Dec. 4, 2001.

Hospital Admission

Marshall LM and Maclennan JG. Environmental Health in Hospital: A Practical Guide for Hospital Staff, Part I: Pollution Prevention. Canadian Society for Environmental Medicine, 2000 Revised Edition
Marshall LM and Maclennan JG. Environmental Health in Hospital: A Practical Guide for Hospital Staff, Part II: Environment-Sensitive Care. Canadian Society for Environmental Medicine, 2000 Revised Edition

GENERAL

Alternative Medicine: The Definitive Guide, Burton Goldberg Group, Future Medicine Publ., 1995

De Marco, C. *Take Charge of Your Body: A Women's Health Advisor.* The Well Women Press, 1994. P.O. Box 66, Winlaw, B.C. V0G 2J0 Canada

Encyclopaedia of Natural Healing: A Practical Self Help Guide. Alive Books, 1997

Fallon, S. *Nourishing Traditions: The Cookbook that Challenges Politically Correct Nutrition and the Diet Dictocrats,* New Trends Publishing, 1999 (1-877-707-1776)

Gore, A. (Senator). *Earth in the Balance, Ecology and the Human Spirit,* Plume Printing, 1993.

Harr, J. *A Civil Action,* Vintage Books, 1996

Harvard Medical School Books, *Healthy Women, Healthy Lives: A Guide to Preventing Disease from the Landmark Nurses' Health Study,* Simon & Schuster, 2001

Holladay, Ruth and Travis, Nick. *The Body Wrecker, You May Have It and Not Know It,* Amarillo Texas, Don Quixote Publishing Co. Inc., 1981

Kerns, T. *Environmentally Induced Illnesses: Ethics, Risk Assessment and Human Rights,* McFarlan & Co., 2001

Moore, T.J. *Prescription for Disaster: The Hidden Dangers in your Medicine Cabinet,* Simon & Schuster, 1998

Porritt, Jonathon. *Where on Earth Are We Going?* BBC Books, Butler & Tanner Ltd. 1990. ISBN: 0-563-20847-3

Radetsky, P. *Allergic to the Twentieth Century,* Little Brown & Co., 1997

Rogers, S. *Wellness Against All Odds,* Prestige Publishing., 1994

Rogers, S. *Tired or Toxic?,* Prestige Publishing, 1990

Rogers, S. *Pain Free in 6 Weeks,* SK Publishers, 2001

Suzuki, D. and Dressler, H. *Good News For A Change: Hope For A Troubled Planet,* Stoddart, 2002

The Earth Works Group. *50 Simple Things Your Business Can Do to Save the Earth* Earth, Works Press, Inc. Berkley California 1991

Rogers, S. *The EI Syndrome: An Rx for Environmental Illness,* SK Publishing, 1995

Rogers, S., *You Are What You Ate,* Prestige Publishing, 1997

Rona, Z., *Return to the Joy of Health,* Alive Books, 1997

Steingraber, S. *Having Faith,* Perseus, 2001

Hilgers, TW and Stanford JB. "Creighton Model NaProEducation Technology for Avoiding Pregnancy: Use Effectiveness". In: The Journal of Reproductive Medicine, Vol. 43, No. 6, June 1998.

Index

NOTES

NOTES

NOTES

NOTES

NOTES

NOTES